AI in Healthcare

Unlock the power of AI to revolutionize patient care, diagnostics, and healthcare innovation. Essential insights for professionals, students, and decision-makers shaping the future of medicine.

Written by

ERIC LEBOUTHILLIER

AcraSolution | 2025 1st Edition
www.acrasolution.com

Preface

Who this book is for

This book is written for healthcare professionals, medical students, AI enthusiasts, policymakers, and entrepreneurs who want to understand how artificial intelligence is transforming the healthcare industry. Whether you are a clinician seeking practical tools, a researcher exploring AI's potential, or a leader preparing your organization for digital transformation, this book will give you a clear and accessible guide.

What to expect from this book

Readers can expect a structured overview of the most important AI applications in healthcare—covering diagnostics, predictive analytics, medical imaging, drug discovery, robotics, patient engagement, and ethical considerations. You'll gain both technical and non-technical insights, real-world examples, and practical frameworks to evaluate, adopt, and responsibly use AI solutions. By the end, you'll have a strong foundation to make informed decisions, stay competitive, and embrace the future of healthcare powered by AI.

All references to laws, regulations, security standards, or industry guidelines are intended for general awareness only and may not reflect the most current legal developments. This publication is not intended to create, and receipt does not constitute, a client relationship with the author, publisher, or any affiliated entity.

By reading, accessing, or applying the content in this publication, you agree to do so at your own risk. If you do not accept these terms, you are advised to discontinue use of this material immediately.

Table of Contents

CHAPTER 1

Foundations of AI in Healthcare

The Evolution of AI and Machine Learning in Medicine

Artificial Intelligence (AI) in healthcare is not a sudden invention. It is the result of decades of progress in computing, data science, and medical research. To understand where we are today—and where healthcare is headed—it helps to look back at how AI and machine learning entered the medical world, step by step.

Early Experiments: Rules and Logic

The first wave of AI in medicine appeared in the 1960s and 70s. Computers were still limited, but researchers tried to teach them medical reasoning. The most famous early example was **MYCIN**, a system built at Stanford in the 1970s to help doctors identify bacterial infections and recommend antibiotics.

MYCIN used "if-then" rules:

- If a patient had certain symptoms,
- And lab results showed a specific pattern,
- Then the system suggested a likely diagnosis.

While it never became widely used in clinics, MYCIN proved that computers could process medical knowledge in a structured way. This rule-based approach, however, struggled in real-world practice. Medicine is full of exceptions, and hard-coded rules could not adapt to the complexity of human biology.

The Data Explosion: A New Era

By the 1990s and early 2000s, hospitals and clinics started moving from paper records to **electronic health records (EHRs)**. Suddenly, medicine had more data than ever before—lab results, prescriptions, imaging, and patient histories were now digital. This shift laid the foundation for machine learning, which thrives on large datasets.

At the same time, advances in computing power made it possible to process millions of data points quickly. Instead of rules, algorithms could now **learn patterns from the data itself**. For example:

- A machine learning model could learn to predict the risk of diabetes by analyzing thousands of patient records.
- Algorithms could detect patterns in X-rays or CT scans that the human eye might miss.

This marked a turning point: medicine was no longer limited to knowledge written by experts. Computers could now discover relationships hidden inside the data.

Deep Learning and the Imaging Revolution

In the 2010s, a breakthrough called **deep learning** transformed AI in healthcare. Deep learning uses neural networks—algorithms inspired by the brain's structure—that can analyze complex data such as images, speech, or free text.

In radiology, for example, deep learning systems can scan thousands of chest X-rays and learn to recognize signs of pneumonia, cancer, or fractures. In dermatology, algorithms trained on large image databases can identify skin cancers as accurately as expert dermatologists.

The key difference is scale. While a human doctor may see thousands of images in a career, an AI model can learn from millions. This gives it statistical power to recognize subtle details consistently and quickly. Instead of replacing radiologists or dermatologists, AI acts as a **second pair of eyes**—a tool to support faster, more accurate decisions.

Beyond Images: Expanding Applications

AI in healthcare is not limited to imaging. Its use has expanded into several areas:

- **Predictive analytics:** AI models can estimate which patients are at higher risk of heart failure, sepsis, or hospital readmission.
- **Drug discovery:** Algorithms analyze biological data to suggest new drug targets, dramatically speeding up research.
- **Natural language processing (NLP):** AI can read and summarize clinical notes, turning unstructured text into usable insights.
- **Virtual health assistants:** Chatbots and digital tools help answer patient questions, schedule appointments, or provide medication reminders.

These applications show how AI is becoming a central part of everyday healthcare operations, not just research labs.

Current Challenges and Realities

Despite rapid progress, AI in medicine is not flawless. Early excitement sometimes led to unrealistic expectations. For example, some tools performed well in controlled studies but failed in real-world hospitals, where patient populations are more diverse. Data quality, privacy concerns, and integration into existing medical workflows remain significant challenges.

Doctors also worry about "black box" algorithms, where AI provides a result without explaining its reasoning. In healthcare, transparency matters. A doctor needs to know *why* an algorithm suggests a diagnosis before acting on it.

A Continuous Evolution

The story of AI in healthcare is ongoing. From rule-based systems like MYCIN, to machine learning models trained on EHRs, to today's deep learning breakthroughs in imaging, each step built on the one before it. Importantly, AI has moved from being an academic experiment to a real-world tool used in clinics, labs, and hospitals around the world.

What makes this evolution powerful is its direction: AI is becoming more accessible, more accurate, and more integrated into the daily practice of medicine. It is no longer about replacing doctors but about augmenting their capabilities.

Takeaway

AI in healthcare did not appear overnight—it has been decades in the making. From early rule-based systems to today's deep learning applications, each phase has pushed medicine forward by unlocking new ways to process information and detect patterns. The lesson is clear: AI in healthcare is not a static technology but a continuously evolving partner, learning from data and shaping the future of medical care.

Key Concepts: Algorithms, Data, and Neural Networks

Understanding how AI works in healthcare starts with three core building blocks: **algorithms, data, and neural networks**. These concepts sound technical, but at their heart, they explain how computers learn, make predictions, and support doctors in medical decision-making.

Algorithms: The Step-by-Step Instructions

An **algorithm** is simply a set of instructions that tells a computer what to do. In healthcare, algorithms can be very simple or highly complex.

- A simple algorithm might calculate a patient's body mass index (BMI) using weight and height.
- A more advanced algorithm might predict a patient's risk of developing heart disease by analyzing hundreds of variables such as age, blood pressure, cholesterol levels, and family history.

The important point is this: algorithms are the "recipes" that process information and produce outcomes. In medicine, the quality of the algorithm directly affects patient care. If an algorithm is well-designed, it can help detect diseases earlier, suggest better treatment options, and reduce human error.

Data: The Fuel of AI

If algorithms are the recipes, then **data** is the ingredient. Without good data, even the best algorithm cannot perform well.

Healthcare generates massive amounts of data every day:

- Electronic health records with diagnoses, lab tests, and prescriptions.
- Medical imaging such as X-rays, MRIs, and CT scans.
- Wearable devices that track heart rate, blood pressure, and activity.
- Genetic information from DNA sequencing.

AI systems learn patterns by analyzing this data. For example:

- By studying thousands of mammograms, an algorithm can learn to detect early signs of breast cancer.
- By analyzing wearable device data, AI can alert a patient to irregular heart rhythms before they become dangerous.

However, not all data is equal. If the data is incomplete, biased, or inaccurate, the AI model may give unreliable results. This is why hospitals and researchers emphasize **data quality and diversity**—to ensure that AI tools work for all types of patients, not just a limited group.

Neural Networks: Learning Like the Brain

The most advanced form of AI in healthcare comes from **neural networks**, especially **deep learning**. These systems are inspired by how the human brain processes information.

A neural network is made up of layers of "neurons" (mathematical functions) that pass information to each other. Each layer detects increasingly complex features. For example, when analyzing a chest X-ray:

1. The first layer may detect simple edges and shapes.
2. The next layer may recognize structures like ribs or lungs.
3. Deeper layers may identify patterns linked to diseases such as pneumonia or lung cancer.

What makes neural networks powerful is their ability to handle unstructured data like images, sound, and text. Unlike traditional algorithms that rely on pre-set rules, neural networks **learn patterns directly from raw data**. This is why they excel at tasks such as image recognition in radiology or natural language processing of clinical notes.

The Connection Between Them

Algorithms, data, and neural networks are not separate ideas—they work together:

- **Algorithms** provide the logic and structure.
- **Data** supplies the real-world evidence for learning.
- **Neural networks** allow AI to handle complexity that simple algorithms cannot.

For example, in diagnosing diabetic retinopathy from retinal scans:

- Data: thousands of labeled images of healthy and diseased eyes.
- Algorithm: a neural network trained to detect disease-related features.
- Outcome: a system that can identify signs of diabetic retinopathy with accuracy comparable to an eye specialist.

Takeaway

AI in healthcare is built on three pillars: algorithms that define the rules, data that feeds the learning, and neural networks that unlock advanced capabilities. Understanding these concepts makes it clear why AI is so powerful—and why its success depends on the quality of the tools and the information it learns from. Together, they form the foundation of every modern AI application in medicine.

Understanding Healthcare Data: Structured vs. Unstructured

AI in healthcare is only as powerful as the data it works with. To see how AI makes sense of medical information, we need to distinguish between **structured data** and **unstructured data**. These two types form the backbone of digital healthcare, but they are very different in how they are created, stored, and used.

Structured Data: Organized and Easy to Process

Structured data is information stored in a clear, organized format—usually in rows and columns like a spreadsheet or database. It is highly standardized and easy for computers to analyze.

Examples of structured healthcare data include:

- Blood pressure readings (e.g., 120/80 mmHg)
- Lab results (cholesterol level: 180 mg/dL)
- Medication prescriptions (drug name, dose, frequency)
- Age, weight, height, or patient ID numbers

This type of data is **precise and numerical**, which makes it perfect for algorithms. For instance:

- A system predicting the risk of heart disease can quickly process lab values, BMI, and blood pressure.
- Hospitals can track trends, such as the average recovery time for patients after surgery.

Structured data is reliable because it follows strict formats. However, it only captures part of the patient's story.

Unstructured Data: Rich but Messy

Unstructured data is information that does not follow a fixed format. It is harder for computers to read, but it contains valuable clinical insights.

Examples of unstructured healthcare data include:

- Doctor's notes and clinical narratives
- Medical imaging (X-rays, MRIs, ultrasounds)
- Audio files (dictations, patient interviews)
- Free-text patient surveys
- Genomic data

Unstructured data is often where the **context** lives. For example:

- A radiology image may reveal signs of lung disease that numbers alone cannot show.
- A doctor's note may mention lifestyle factors—such as stress, diet, or smoking—that strongly affect health outcomes but are not stored in structured fields.

This kind of data is rich but messy. Without AI, it is almost impossible to process at scale.

How AI Brings Structure to the Unstructured

This is where AI, especially **natural language processing (NLP)** and **computer vision**, becomes essential:

- NLP tools can read free-text clinical notes, pull out key information, and turn it into structured data. For example, if a note says "patient has a history of hypertension," AI can convert that into a structured diagnosis field.
- Computer vision algorithms can analyze imaging data, highlight abnormalities, and even quantify measurements like tumor size.

By transforming unstructured data into usable insights, AI expands the amount of knowledge doctors can access without overwhelming them.

Why the Difference Matters

Understanding structured vs. unstructured data is not just technical—it affects patient care directly. For example:

- If a hospital only looks at structured data, it may miss critical insights buried in doctors' notes or imaging results.
- If AI tools can combine both types of data, predictions become far more accurate. A cancer diagnosis, for instance,

may depend not just on lab values (structured) but also on MRI scans and biopsy reports (unstructured).

Takeaway

Healthcare data comes in two forms: structured, which is clean and easy for computers to process, and unstructured, which is complex but full of hidden value. The future of AI in medicine lies in bringing these two worlds together—turning raw, unstructured information into structured knowledge that improves diagnosis, treatment, and patient outcomes.

Opportunities and Limitations of AI Adoption in Healthcare

AI is transforming healthcare, but it is not a magic cure. Its power lies in its ability to analyze vast amounts of information, detect patterns, and support medical decision-making. At the same time, there are real limitations that must be addressed before AI can fully deliver on its promise. Understanding both sides—opportunities and challenges—helps us see how AI can be applied responsibly.

Opportunities: Where AI Adds Value

AI opens new possibilities across almost every corner of healthcare.

1. Early Disease Detection
AI can spot signs of disease earlier than the human eye. For example:

- Algorithms can detect diabetic retinopathy from retinal scans before vision loss occurs.
- AI can flag suspicious lung nodules in CT scans, allowing cancer to be treated at earlier stages.

Early detection saves lives and reduces treatment costs.

2. Personalized Medicine
AI can analyze genetic data, lifestyle factors, and medical history to tailor treatment to individual patients. Instead of "one-size-fits-all" care, doctors can recommend therapies more likely to work for each person.

3. Operational Efficiency
Hospitals generate huge administrative burdens—scheduling, billing, and paperwork. AI can automate many of these tasks, freeing up time for doctors and nurses to focus on patients.

4. Predictive Analytics
AI systems can forecast which patients are at risk of complications. For example:

- Predicting which patients might develop sepsis in intensive care.
- Identifying those likely to be readmitted after surgery.

This allows preventive action before a crisis develops.

5. Accelerated Drug Discovery
Traditional drug development takes years and costs billions. AI can analyze chemical structures, simulate interactions, and suggest promising compounds, significantly speeding up research.

Limitations: The Barriers to Widespread Use

Despite its potential, AI adoption in healthcare faces important challenges.

1. Data Quality and Bias
AI models are only as good as the data they are trained on. If the data is incomplete or biased, the results will be flawed. For instance, an algorithm trained mostly on data from one ethnic group may not perform well on others.

2. Integration with Clinical Workflows

Healthcare is complex, and doctors cannot afford to work with tools that slow them down. If AI systems are not smoothly integrated into existing workflows, they may go unused.

3. Transparency and Trust

Many AI systems function as "black boxes," giving answers without clear explanations. Doctors need to understand *why* an AI suggests a diagnosis or treatment before they can trust it. Lack of transparency slows adoption.

4. Regulatory and Legal Issues

Healthcare is heavily regulated for good reason. AI tools must be proven safe and effective before they are approved for use. There are also legal questions: if an AI makes a mistake, who is responsible— the developer, the hospital, or the doctor?

5. Privacy Concerns

Medical data is highly sensitive. Using it to train AI raises concerns about patient privacy and data security. Hospitals must balance innovation with strict protection of personal health information.

Striking the Balance

AI in healthcare is not about replacing doctors but enhancing their abilities. It is most effective when used as a **decision-support tool**, giving doctors additional insights without taking away their judgment. The challenge is building systems that are accurate, fair, explainable, and practical in real-world clinical settings.

Takeaway

AI offers healthcare enormous opportunities: faster diagnosis, personalized care, efficient operations, predictive insights, and faster drug discovery. At the same time, adoption is limited by issues of data quality, bias, integration, trust, regulation, and privacy. Growth will come from balancing these strengths and weaknesses— leveraging AI's potential while carefully managing its risks.

CHAPTER 2

AI in Diagnostics and Imaging

Computer Vision for X-rays, CT, and MRI Scans

Medical imaging is one of the most successful areas of AI in healthcare. Every day, millions of X-rays, CT scans, and MRI scans are taken worldwide. Traditionally, radiologists analyze these images to detect fractures, tumors, infections, or other abnormalities. But with the growing demand for imaging and a shortage of specialists, radiologists are under pressure. This is where **computer vision**, a branch of AI that allows machines to "see" and interpret images, is making a major impact.

Why Imaging Needs AI

Radiologists often review hundreds of images daily. Even for experts, this level of workload can lead to fatigue and the risk of missed findings. Medical images are also increasingly detailed; a single CT scan can contain hundreds of slices, each requiring careful review.

AI-powered computer vision systems help by:

- **Prioritizing urgent cases** (e.g., detecting a brain hemorrhage and alerting doctors immediately).
- **Highlighting suspicious regions** on images for closer inspection.
- **Providing a second opinion** to reduce human error.

The goal is not to replace radiologists but to give them a reliable assistant that works tirelessly, without fatigue.

X-rays: Quick and Widespread

X-rays are the most common imaging test, used for conditions like broken bones, lung infections, and heart enlargement. AI algorithms can now:

- Detect **pneumonia** on chest X-rays with accuracy similar to radiologists.
- Identify **fractures** in bones that might be missed in busy emergency rooms.
- Monitor **tuberculosis** in areas where radiologists are scarce.

For instance, in rural clinics, AI systems integrated into X-ray machines can give instant results, helping doctors make quicker decisions when specialists are not available.

CT Scans: Layer by Layer Analysis

CT (computed tomography) scans provide more detail than X-rays, creating cross-sectional images of the body. They are crucial for detecting cancers, strokes, and internal injuries.

AI in CT analysis is being used to:

- Spot **early lung nodules**, which may signal lung cancer.
- Detect **strokes** by identifying blocked or bleeding blood vessels in the brain.
- Assess **COVID-19 severity** by measuring lung involvement.

Because CT scans generate hundreds of slices, AI's ability to quickly process and highlight abnormalities reduces the burden on radiologists while increasing accuracy.

MRI Scans: Complex but Insightful

MRI (magnetic resonance imaging) provides highly detailed images of soft tissues such as the brain, spinal cord, and joints. MRIs take longer to perform and produce more complex data, which can delay diagnosis.

AI helps in MRI by:

- Accelerating scan reconstruction, making imaging faster and more comfortable for patients.
- Detecting subtle changes in brain tissue that may indicate early **Alzheimer's disease** or **multiple sclerosis**.
- Measuring tumor size and response to treatment with precision.

These capabilities allow for earlier intervention and better tracking of disease progression.

Strengths and Challenges

The strengths of computer vision in imaging are clear: faster interpretation, greater accuracy, and improved access in areas with few specialists. However, challenges remain:

- AI may perform well on training data but struggle with images from different machines or populations.
- False positives can overwhelm doctors with unnecessary alerts.
- Regulatory approval and integration into hospital systems take time.

Takeaway

Computer vision is revolutionizing diagnostics by turning X-rays, CTs, and MRIs into powerful sources of AI-driven insight. From detecting pneumonia in rural clinics to flagging strokes in emergency settings, AI acts as a safety net for radiologists and patients alike. Its greatest value is not in replacing specialists but in ensuring that no critical detail is overlooked.

Early Disease Detection Through Predictive Models

One of the biggest advantages of AI in medicine is its ability to detect diseases before symptoms become obvious. Traditionally, many illnesses are diagnosed only after they have progressed—sometimes too far for effective treatment. Predictive models powered by AI are changing this by analyzing patterns in patient data and flagging risks early.

The Shift From Reactive to Proactive Medicine

Healthcare has long been **reactive**: doctors treat patients after they fall sick. Predictive models move medicine toward a **proactive** approach. Instead of waiting for symptoms, AI uses available data—lab tests, imaging, genetic information, and lifestyle records—to estimate the likelihood of future disease.

This shift means:

- **Earlier intervention** (e.g., lifestyle changes or preventive drugs).
- **Better outcomes** because treatment starts before the disease advances.
- **Reduced costs** since preventing illness is cheaper than treating it later.

How Predictive Models Work

At the core, predictive models use historical patient data to learn patterns linked to disease. Once trained, they can assess new patients and estimate their risk.

For example:

- A model might analyze blood sugar levels, weight, and activity patterns to predict **diabetes risk**.
- Another might use genetic markers and family history to forecast **breast cancer susceptibility**.
- Hospital-based models can combine lab values and vital signs to predict **sepsis**, often hours before symptoms become obvious.

What makes AI powerful is its ability to integrate **hundreds of factors at once**, something humans cannot do efficiently.

Real-World Applications

1. Cardiovascular Disease
AI systems can predict heart attacks by analyzing ECG patterns, cholesterol levels, and lifestyle data. In some studies, algorithms spotted heart problems earlier than standard clinical methods.

2. Cancer
Predictive models trained on imaging and genetic data can flag patients likely to develop cancer before a tumor even appears. For instance, AI tools analyzing mammograms have been shown to predict breast cancer risk up to five years in advance.

3. Neurological Disorders
Early detection of Alzheimer's disease or Parkinson's is difficult with traditional methods. AI can analyze subtle changes in brain scans or speech patterns, signaling disease years before clinical diagnosis.

4. Infectious Diseases
During the COVID-19 pandemic, predictive models were used to identify patients at risk of severe illness, helping hospitals allocate resources and prioritize care.

Challenges of Predictive Medicine

Despite its promise, predictive modeling comes with challenges:

- **False positives:** Over-predicting disease risk may cause unnecessary anxiety or treatment.
- **Bias in data:** If models are trained mostly on one population group, predictions may not generalize well to others.
- **Ethical concerns:** Predicting disease raises sensitive questions—how should patients be informed about risks they might never develop?
- **Integration into care:** Doctors must balance AI predictions with medical judgment, avoiding over-reliance on algorithms.

Takeaway

Predictive models represent a shift from treating disease to **preventing it**. By analyzing patient data, AI can identify risks for heart disease, cancer, dementia, and more—often years before symptoms appear. While challenges of accuracy, bias, and ethics remain, the potential is transformative: saving lives through early detection and empowering patients with knowledge before illness takes hold.

AI-Powered Pathology and Laboratory Analysis

Pathology and laboratory testing are the foundation of modern medicine. From blood counts to tissue biopsies, lab results guide most clinical decisions. Traditionally, pathologists and lab technicians rely on microscopes and manual analysis. With AI, this process is being transformed—making diagnostics faster, more accurate, and more scalable.

Why Pathology Matters

Pathology is about understanding disease at its root. A single tissue sample can reveal whether a tumor is benign or malignant, and a blood test can show early signs of infection or organ damage. However, these tasks are highly labor-intensive:

- Pathologists often review **hundreds of slides** a week.
- Lab technicians process **thousands of samples** daily.
- Small human errors can have large consequences for patients.

AI offers a way to ease this workload while enhancing precision.

Digital Pathology Meets AI

Traditionally, pathology slides are viewed under microscopes. Now, many labs are adopting **digital pathology**, where slides are scanned into high-resolution images. These images can then be analyzed by AI systems.

AI in pathology can:

- Detect cancerous cells in biopsy samples.
- Classify tumor types and grade their severity.
- Quantify features like tumor size or spread.

For example, in breast cancer biopsies, AI can highlight suspicious areas, ensuring pathologists don't miss small clusters of malignant cells. This acts as a safety net while also speeding up diagnosis.

AI in Laboratory Analysis

Beyond pathology, AI is also reshaping general laboratory medicine. Labs generate vast amounts of structured data—blood counts, enzyme levels, hormone assays, genetic tests.

AI can process this data to:

- Flag abnormal results instantly for urgent review.
- Correlate test patterns with potential diseases.
- Predict complications by combining multiple test results over time.

For example:

- AI can analyze **complete blood counts** to predict early signs of leukemia.
- In microbiology labs, AI tools can identify bacteria from culture images, reducing turnaround time for infection diagnosis.
- In genomics, AI helps identify disease-causing mutations from billions of DNA sequences.

Speed and Scale

One of AI's biggest advantages in labs is **scalability**. While a human pathologist can only analyze a limited number of slides per day, AI can screen thousands. This is particularly valuable in regions with **shortages of specialists**. AI can handle the first review, flagging slides for closer human inspection.

Challenges to Overcome

Despite its promise, AI-powered pathology and lab analysis face barriers:

- **Standardization issues:** Slide preparation and staining methods vary across labs, which can affect AI accuracy.
- **Data requirements:** High-quality labeled images are needed to train models, and building these datasets takes time.
- **Regulation and validation:** AI tools must undergo rigorous testing before they are trusted in clinical workflows.

- **Acceptance by specialists:** Pathologists must feel AI supports, not replaces, their expertise.

Takeaway

AI is transforming pathology and laboratory analysis from manual, time-consuming processes into faster, more precise systems. By analyzing digital slides, lab data, and genetic information, AI helps pathologists detect disease earlier and with greater accuracy. The future is not about replacing human experts but about giving them tools to handle rising demand while ensuring no critical detail is overlooked.

Case Studies: Reducing Diagnostic Errors with AI

Diagnostic errors are among the most serious challenges in healthcare. According to studies, millions of patients worldwide are affected each year by delayed or incorrect diagnoses. These errors can lead to unnecessary treatments, worsened outcomes, or even preventable deaths. AI is emerging as a key tool to reduce such errors by acting as a second layer of review, catching patterns that humans may overlook.

Case Study 1: Detecting Lung Cancer from CT Scans

In lung cancer, early detection is critical. Yet, small nodules on CT scans are easy to miss, especially when radiologists must review hundreds of images in a single scan. Google Health researchers developed a deep learning model trained on thousands of CT scans.

Result:

- The AI system outperformed six experienced radiologists in detecting lung cancer nodules.
- It reduced both false negatives (missed cancers) and false positives (unnecessary follow-ups).

This case shows how AI can provide a safety net, ensuring fewer cancers slip through unnoticed.

Case Study 2: Preventing Misdiagnosis in Diabetic Retinopathy

Diabetic retinopathy is a leading cause of blindness. Many patients in rural or low-resource areas do not have access to eye specialists, leading to late diagnoses. AI-based retinal screening systems have been deployed in clinics across India and Thailand.

Result:

- AI analyzed retinal images instantly, flagging high-risk cases for referral.
- This reduced delays in diagnosis and ensured patients received timely treatment.

Here, AI closed the gap where specialists were unavailable, directly preventing diagnostic errors of omission.

Case Study 3: Identifying Breast Cancer from Mammograms

Traditional mammogram interpretation has a significant error rate— both missed cancers and unnecessary recalls. A study in the UK tested an AI system on over 25,000 mammograms.

Result:

- The AI matched the accuracy of expert radiologists.
- When used together with human review, diagnostic errors were reduced by nearly 20%.

This illustrates the value of **AI as a partner**, not a replacement, providing double-checking capabilities that reduce mistakes.

Case Study 4: Sepsis Prediction in Hospitals

Sepsis, a life-threatening complication of infection, is often missed in its early stages because symptoms overlap with other conditions. Hospitals in the US have tested AI models that continuously monitor patient vitals and lab data.

Result:

- The AI flagged sepsis risk hours before clinicians recognized it.
- Early alerts allowed faster treatment, significantly lowering mortality rates.

This case highlights how AI reduces diagnostic delays in fast-moving emergencies where every hour counts.

Lessons Learned from the Cases

Across these examples, a pattern emerges:

- AI reduces errors by **providing an additional safety layer**.
- It excels in handling **large volumes of data** that overwhelm human attention.
- Success is highest when AI is integrated into workflows as a **support tool**, not as a stand-alone replacement for doctors.

Takeaway

Case studies from lung cancer, diabetic retinopathy, breast cancer, and sepsis show that AI is already reducing diagnostic errors in real-world settings. Its value lies in early detection, consistency, and acting as a partner to healthcare professionals. The evidence is clear: AI is not a theoretical tool but a proven technology that saves lives by preventing the errors humans alone cannot always avoid.

CHAPTER 3

Personalized Medicine and Patient Care

Genomics and AI-Driven Treatment Plans

Personalized medicine is based on the idea that treatment should be tailored to the individual, not just the disease. Genomics—the study of a person's DNA—plays a central role in this approach. Our genes influence how we respond to medications, our risk of developing certain conditions, and even how diseases progress. The challenge is that genomic data is massive and complex. This is where AI becomes essential: it can process billions of data points and translate genetic information into actionable treatment plans.

Why Genomics Matters

Every human genome contains over **3 billion DNA bases**. Hidden within this code are variations that can increase the risk of diseases such as cancer, diabetes, or heart disease. Genomics allows doctors to:

- Identify inherited risks (e.g., BRCA mutations linked to breast cancer).
- Predict how a patient might respond to specific drugs.
- Guide preventive care based on genetic predispositions.

However, analyzing raw DNA sequences is like trying to read the world's largest instruction manual in a foreign language. AI helps decode this complexity.

AI in Genomic Analysis

AI algorithms can scan through massive genetic datasets quickly, identifying patterns that humans cannot. Applications include:

- **Variant detection:** AI pinpoints specific mutations that may cause disease.
- **Gene-disease mapping:** Algorithms link genetic variations to known conditions.

- **Pharmacogenomics:** AI predicts how a patient will respond to a medication, reducing trial-and-error in prescribing.

For example, instead of giving all cancer patients the same chemotherapy, AI can help determine which drug combination is most likely to work based on the patient's tumor genetics.

AI-Driven Treatment Plans

When genomic insights are combined with AI, doctors can design treatment plans that are **highly personalized**.

- In oncology, AI-powered systems recommend therapies targeted to the unique mutations in a patient's tumor.
- In cardiology, genetic data combined with AI can predict risk for heart rhythm disorders, guiding preventive treatment.
- In rare diseases, where patients often wait years for a diagnosis, AI can match genetic patterns to known disease profiles, accelerating both diagnosis and treatment.

This approach shifts medicine away from population averages toward truly **individualized care**.

Real-World Impact

A few real-world examples illustrate this transformation:

- **IBM Watson for Oncology** has been tested in cancer care, where it suggests treatment options based on both medical literature and the patient's genetic profile.
- **Deep learning models in genomics** have identified new drug targets by analyzing complex DNA sequences, speeding up drug discovery.
- Hospitals are increasingly using AI tools to integrate genomic data into electronic health records, allowing real-time decision support for clinicians.

Challenges Ahead

While promising, AI in genomics faces hurdles:

- **Data privacy:** Genomic data is deeply personal, raising security concerns.
- **Interpretation gaps:** Not all genetic variants have clear meanings, and AI can suggest links that require further validation.
- **Equity issues:** Most genomic databases are based on European populations, creating risks of bias when applied to diverse groups.

Overcoming these challenges will be critical to making AI-driven genomics useful for everyone.

Takeaway

Genomics unlocks the blueprint of human health, and AI provides the tools to interpret it at scale. Together, they enable treatment plans that are more precise, more effective, and more personal than ever before. While challenges of privacy, interpretation, and equity remain, the integration of AI and genomics is moving us closer to a world where medicine is not just about treating disease, but about tailoring care to each unique patient.

Wearables and Continuous Health Monitoring

Healthcare no longer happens only inside hospitals and clinics. With the rise of wearable devices—such as smartwatches, fitness trackers, and connected sensors—patients can now monitor their health in real time. When combined with AI, these devices do more than just count steps; they can detect early warning signs, support chronic disease management, and empower patients to take control of their own health.

From Fitness Tracking to Medical Monitoring

The first wave of wearables focused on lifestyle metrics: steps walked, calories burned, or hours of sleep. These consumer devices laid the foundation for medical-grade monitoring. Now, advanced wearables can track:

- **Heart rate and rhythm** (detecting irregularities like atrial fibrillation).
- **Blood oxygen levels** (useful for lung conditions and sleep apnea).
- **Blood pressure and glucose** (essential for managing hypertension and diabetes).
- **Activity and mobility** (helpful in monitoring recovery after surgery or injury).

The shift is clear: wearables are evolving from **wellness tools** into **clinical devices**.

AI's Role in Continuous Monitoring

AI enhances wearables by analyzing streams of data and turning them into actionable insights. Continuous monitoring generates millions of data points, far too many for doctors to review manually. AI systems can:

- Detect abnormal patterns in real time and send alerts.
- Predict health risks before symptoms appear.
- Personalize recommendations based on individual baselines rather than general averages.

For example, if a wearable detects unusual heart rhythms, AI can determine whether it's a harmless variation or a sign of atrial fibrillation that requires medical attention.

Real-World Applications

1. Cardiac Care
Apple Watch and similar devices have FDA-approved features for detecting atrial fibrillation. Studies show these alerts have led users to seek care early, preventing strokes.

2. Diabetes Management
Continuous glucose monitors (CGMs) paired with AI can recommend insulin doses, diet adjustments, or activity changes in real time. This is life-changing for patients with type 1 diabetes.

3. Post-Surgery Recovery
Wearables track mobility and vital signs after surgery, allowing doctors to monitor recovery remotely and intervene early if complications arise.

4. Mental Health and Stress
AI systems analyze sleep quality, heart rate variability, and activity patterns to detect stress, anxiety, or depression risk, supporting early mental health interventions.

Empowering Patients

One of the most significant impacts of wearables is **patient empowerment**. Instead of relying only on occasional doctor visits, patients gain a continuous view of their health. This encourages healthier habits and improves adherence to treatment plans.

For instance, a patient with hypertension can see how diet, exercise, or medication changes affect blood pressure in real time—making health management more tangible and motivating.

Challenges of Wearable Technology

Despite the promise, challenges remain:

- **Data overload:** Too many alerts can overwhelm both patients and doctors.
- **Accuracy concerns:** Consumer-grade devices may not always match medical-grade precision.
- **Privacy risks:** Continuous data collection raises questions about how health data is stored and shared.
- **Accessibility:** Not all patients can afford or use advanced wearables, creating inequalities in access.

Takeaway

Wearables, powered by AI, are shifting healthcare from the clinic to the wrist, offering continuous monitoring and real-time insights. From detecting heart conditions to managing diabetes, these tools enable earlier interventions and empower patients to take an active role in their care. While accuracy, privacy, and equity must be addressed, the integration of wearables into everyday life signals a future where healthcare is personalized, proactive, and always within reach.

AI for Mental Health and Behavioral Analysis

Mental health is one of the most pressing healthcare challenges today. Conditions such as depression, anxiety, and burnout affect millions worldwide, yet diagnosis often relies on self-reporting and limited face-to-face interactions with clinicians. Unlike physical illnesses, mental health disorders can remain invisible until they become severe. AI offers new ways to detect, monitor, and support mental health by analyzing behavior, speech, and digital patterns that are difficult for humans to track at scale.

Why Mental Health Needs AI

Traditional mental health care faces several barriers:

- **Stigma** prevents many from seeking help.
- **Shortages of specialists** mean long wait times.
- **Subjective assessments** can miss early warning signs.

AI helps address these gaps by providing **objective, continuous, and scalable monitoring**. It doesn't replace therapists but offers tools to reach more patients earlier.

Behavioral and Speech Analysis

AI systems can analyze subtle behavioral changes that indicate shifts in mental health. Examples include:

- **Voice patterns:** Depression and anxiety can affect tone, pitch, and speech pace. AI can detect these variations during phone calls or therapy sessions.
- **Facial expressions and movement:** Computer vision can identify micro-expressions or reduced activity linked to mood disorders.
- **Digital behavior:** Changes in texting frequency, sleep tracked via wearables, or reduced social interaction online can signal declining mental well-being.

These insights allow earlier intervention, often before the person themselves recognizes the problem.

Chatbots and Virtual Therapists

AI-powered chatbots provide **24/7 conversational support**, making mental health care more accessible. Tools like Woebot or Wysa engage users in cognitive-behavioral therapy (CBT) techniques through simple text or voice interactions.

Benefits include:

- Immediate emotional support in moments of stress.
- Nonjudgmental conversations, reducing stigma.
- Guidance on coping strategies, mindfulness, and daily routines.

While they cannot replace human therapists, they serve as valuable companions between therapy sessions or for those with limited access to care.

Predictive Mental Health Models

AI also predicts **risk of crises** by analyzing data streams:

- Wearables can track sleep, heart rate variability, and activity to flag signs of burnout or depression.
- Algorithms analyzing medical and social data can identify patients at risk of suicide, enabling timely outreach.
- In workplace wellness programs, AI tools help employers detect stress trends while protecting individual privacy.

Challenges and Ethical Questions

Mental health AI comes with sensitive concerns:

- **Privacy:** Behavioral and emotional data are deeply personal, requiring strict safeguards.
- **False positives:** Over-alerting can cause unnecessary worry or overwhelm providers.
- **Trust:** Patients may feel uneasy about machines analyzing their moods.
- **Human touch:** AI cannot replace empathy and the therapeutic relationship essential for healing.

Takeaway

AI is reshaping mental health care by detecting subtle behavioral signals, offering on-demand chatbot support, and predicting risks before crises occur. While it cannot replace human therapists, it expands access, reduces stigma, and enables early intervention. The future of mental health care may be hybrid—where AI handles monitoring and routine support, while human professionals focus on empathy, understanding, and deeper therapeutic care.

Improving Patient Outcomes with Precision Care

The ultimate goal of personalized medicine is to improve patient outcomes—not just to treat disease, but to treat the *right patient with the right intervention at the right time*. Precision care combines genomics, wearable data, predictive models, and AI-driven insights to move beyond averages and design treatments tailored to individuals. This shift is already transforming survival rates, quality of life, and overall healthcare efficiency.

From One-Size-Fits-All to Tailored Interventions

Traditional medicine often takes a standardized approach: the same drug, dosage, or therapy is given to large groups of patients. While effective for some, this approach leaves many without optimal results. Precision care, powered by AI, changes this by:

- Identifying which patients will benefit from a specific treatment.
- Predicting side effects based on genetic or lifestyle factors.
- Adjusting care dynamically as the patient's condition evolves.

For example, in oncology, two patients with the same type of cancer may respond very differently to the same chemotherapy. AI can analyze genetic profiles and tumor biology to recommend **targeted therapies** that maximize effectiveness and minimize harm.

AI's Role in Precision Care

AI integrates diverse data sources—genomic sequencing, imaging, lab results, and wearable sensors—to create a **comprehensive patient profile**. With this, AI can:

- Recommend the most effective drug combinations.
- Suggest lifestyle interventions that align with the patient's unique risks.
- Monitor patient response in real time and adjust treatment plans automatically.

Instead of static care plans, precision medicine supported by AI enables **dynamic, personalized care pathways**.

Real-World Impact

1. Oncology
AI-driven platforms analyze tumor DNA to match patients with targeted drugs or immunotherapies. Some cancer centers are already using these tools to increase survival rates and reduce unnecessary treatments.

2. Cardiology
AI predicts which heart failure patients are most at risk of hospitalization. Precision interventions—adjusting medications, lifestyle coaching, or remote monitoring—reduce hospital readmissions.

3. Diabetes
AI-powered insulin dosing systems connected to continuous glucose monitors help patients maintain tighter glucose control, reducing long-term complications.

4. Rare Diseases
For conditions often misdiagnosed for years, AI compares patient genetic data to global databases, dramatically accelerating time to treatment.

Benefits for Patients and Providers

Precision care improves outcomes in multiple ways:

- **Better survival and recovery rates** through earlier, more accurate interventions.
- **Reduced side effects** by avoiding ineffective or harmful treatments.
- **Higher patient engagement** since care feels personal and relevant.
- **Cost savings** by targeting resources where they have the greatest impact.

Doctors also benefit from having AI-driven decision support, reducing uncertainty in complex cases.

Challenges to Precision Care

To fully realize its potential, precision care must overcome key barriers:

- **Data integration:** Combining genomics, wearables, and clinical records into one system is technically complex.
- **Equity:** Access to advanced genetic testing and AI tools is not equal worldwide.
- **Clinical adoption:** Doctors need training and confidence in AI-supported recommendations.

- **Ethical questions:** Personalizing care at the genetic level raises concerns about privacy and potential misuse.

Takeaway

Precision care, enabled by AI, represents a leap forward in healthcare. By moving beyond averages and tailoring treatment to individuals, it improves survival, reduces side effects, and empowers patients to take part in their health journey. The vision is clear: a future where every patient receives care that is not just standard, but *precisely theirs*.

CHAPTER 4

AI in Clinical Operations and Workflow

Automating Administrative Tasks and Medical Records

Behind every doctor's visit lies a mountain of paperwork. From entering patient notes to processing insurance claims, administrative work consumes a large share of healthcare resources. In fact, studies show that doctors often spend as much—or more—time on documentation as they do with patients. This not only creates frustration for clinicians but also slows down the entire healthcare system. AI is stepping in to ease this burden, streamlining administrative tasks and transforming how medical records are managed.

The Administrative Challenge in Healthcare

Administrative inefficiency is a global issue:

- Doctors spend hours entering notes into **electronic health records (EHRs)**.
- Nurses and staff juggle scheduling, billing, and insurance verification.
- Errors in coding or incomplete documentation lead to claim rejections and financial losses.

These tasks are necessary but often **pull clinicians away from direct patient care**. Automating them with AI has the potential to free up time, reduce errors, and lower costs.

AI in Medical Documentation

One of the most promising applications of AI is in **clinical documentation**. Tools using **natural language processing (NLP)** can:

- Convert spoken conversations between doctor and patient into structured medical notes.

- Extract key details (diagnoses, prescriptions, symptoms) from free-text notes.
- Suggest coding for billing and insurance purposes automatically.

For example, AI-powered "medical scribes" listen to consultations and generate accurate notes, which doctors can review and sign off within minutes. This reduces paperwork and allows physicians to focus fully on their patients during visits.

Automating Medical Records Management

AI also improves how medical records are stored and retrieved. Traditional EHRs are often cluttered and difficult to navigate. AI-driven systems can:

- Summarize a patient's history into a **clear, concise overview**.
- Highlight critical changes in lab results or imaging over time.
- Identify missing information and prompt clinicians to complete records.

This means doctors spend less time searching for details and more time making informed decisions.

Administrative Process Automation

Beyond records, AI is reshaping other administrative workflows:

- **Scheduling:** AI predicts no-shows and optimizes appointment times.
- **Billing and coding:** Algorithms review medical charts and assign accurate codes, reducing claim denials.
- **Insurance claims:** AI systems can auto-verify eligibility and speed up approvals.
- **Supply chain management:** Predictive models ensure hospitals maintain the right levels of medication and equipment.

Together, these automations reduce bottlenecks, lower costs, and improve patient flow.

Benefits for Clinicians and Patients

The benefits of automating administrative tasks extend beyond efficiency:

- Clinicians regain time for patient care.
- Hospitals save money by reducing errors and speeding up workflows.
- Patients experience shorter wait times, fewer billing issues, and smoother communication.

When done well, automation improves both the **experience of care** and the **quality of care**.

Challenges to Overcome

Despite the promise, several challenges exist:

- **Data security:** Automating sensitive records increases the risk of breaches.
- **System compatibility:** Many hospitals use outdated EHR systems that are hard to integrate with AI.
- **Accuracy:** Errors in automated coding or transcription must be carefully monitored.
- **Adoption resistance:** Some clinicians are hesitant to trust AI with critical documentation tasks.

Takeaway

AI is lifting the burden of administrative work in healthcare by automating documentation, streamlining medical records, and optimizing workflows like billing and scheduling. The result is more time for clinicians to focus on patients and a more efficient healthcare system overall. While challenges of security, integration, and trust remain, the trend is clear: automation is not just about efficiency—it's about bringing healthcare back to its true focus, the patient.

AI-Driven Triage and Patient Scheduling

One of the biggest challenges in healthcare operations is making sure patients are seen at the right time by the right provider. Emergency rooms often face overcrowding, clinics deal with long wait times, and specialists struggle to manage referrals efficiently. Mismanaged scheduling doesn't just cause frustration—it can delay care and worsen outcomes. AI is being applied to triage and scheduling to optimize how patients move through the healthcare system, ensuring faster, fairer, and more efficient access to care.

The Problem of Traditional Triage and Scheduling

In most hospitals and clinics, triage and scheduling are still manual:

- Nurses or staff rely on quick judgment to decide which patient needs urgent attention.
- Appointment slots are fixed, without flexibility for emergencies or cancellations.
- Administrative staff often have limited visibility into overall patient flow, leading to bottlenecks.

This results in **overcrowded emergency rooms, missed appointments**, and uneven distribution of workload among providers.

AI in Patient Triage

AI-powered triage tools use clinical data and patient-reported symptoms to prioritize care.

These systems can:

- Analyze vital signs and lab results to flag high-risk cases (e.g., potential sepsis or stroke).
- Sort patients into urgency levels in emergency departments.
- Support telehealth by guiding patients to the right care setting—emergency, urgent care, or primary care.

For example, smartphone-based triage apps allow patients to enter their symptoms. AI then determines whether they can manage at home, see a doctor, or go to the emergency department immediately. This reduces unnecessary ER visits and ensures critical cases are not delayed.

AI in Scheduling

Scheduling is another area where inefficiency is common. Patients wait weeks for appointments, while providers often face last-minute cancellations that waste valuable time. AI-driven scheduling tools address these problems by:

- **Predicting no-shows** and overbooking strategically to reduce wasted slots.
- **Matching patients with providers** based on condition, availability, and urgency.
- **Dynamic rescheduling** when cancellations occur, automatically filling open slots.
- **Coordinating across departments**, ensuring imaging, lab tests, and consultations align efficiently.

For instance, a hospital AI scheduling system may recognize that a patient with chest pain needs both a cardiology appointment and an imaging test. Instead of scheduling these separately, the system coordinates them in a single streamlined visit.

Real-World Impact

Hospitals using AI-driven scheduling report:

- **Shorter wait times** for patients.
- **Higher efficiency** in using provider time and hospital resources.
- **Better patient satisfaction**, as care feels more coordinated and responsive.

During the COVID-19 pandemic, AI-based triage systems helped hospitals allocate limited ICU beds and ventilators, ensuring resources went to patients most likely to benefit.

Challenges to Adoption

Despite the benefits, challenges remain:

- **Accuracy of AI triage**: Misclassification could delay urgent care or overwhelm emergency services with false alarms.
- **Patient trust**: Some patients may resist AI systems making decisions about urgency.
- **Integration issues**: Scheduling systems must work seamlessly with existing hospital software.
- **Equity concerns**: AI trained on biased data may prioritize care unfairly.

Takeaway

AI-driven triage and scheduling bring order to one of healthcare's most chaotic areas: patient flow. By predicting urgency, reducing no-shows, and dynamically managing appointments, AI ensures patients receive care when they need it while maximizing the efficiency of healthcare providers. The result is faster treatment, reduced delays, and better use of hospital resources—a win for both patients and the system.

Virtual Assistants for Clinicians and Patients

AI-powered virtual assistants are becoming essential tools in healthcare. These systems use natural language processing, machine learning, and voice recognition to help both clinicians and patients manage information, make decisions, and save time. Unlike generic chatbots, medical virtual assistants are designed with healthcare-specific knowledge, allowing them to perform meaningful tasks in clinical and patient-facing settings.

Virtual Assistants for Clinicians

Doctors and nurses often face information overload—thousands of pages of medical guidelines, patient histories scattered across records, and long administrative lists. Virtual assistants reduce this burden by:

- **Retrieving patient data quickly**: A doctor can ask, "What were this patient's last three blood pressure readings?" and get an instant response.
- **Voice-based documentation**: Clinicians dictate notes, and the assistant automatically structures them into the patient's electronic record.
- **Clinical decision support**: Virtual assistants can surface relevant guidelines, suggest possible diagnoses, or flag drug interactions.
- **Task automation**: From ordering lab tests to scheduling follow-up visits, assistants handle routine actions in the background.

This means clinicians spend less time navigating software and more time focusing on patient care.

Virtual Assistants for Patients

Patients often leave clinics with limited recall of instructions and questions that arise later. Virtual assistants bridge this gap by providing continuous support outside the hospital or doctor's office. Common uses include:

- **Medication reminders**: Alerts to take drugs at the right time and dosage.
- **Symptom tracking**: Patients report daily updates (e.g., pain levels, blood sugar) which the assistant monitors for concerning changes.
- **Appointment management**: Scheduling, rescheduling, and sending reminders automatically.
- **Health education**: Explaining conditions, test results, or recovery steps in simple, accessible language.

In chronic disease management, assistants act like a "digital coach," encouraging adherence to treatment and healthy habits.

Real-World Examples

- **Suki AI**: A voice-enabled assistant for doctors that reduces time spent on clinical notes.
- **Sensely**: A patient-facing assistant that helps check symptoms and guide users to appropriate care.
- **Hospital chatbots**: Used during the COVID-19 pandemic to screen symptoms, answer FAQs, and reduce pressure on call centers.

These tools are already showing measurable benefits: reduced clinician burnout, improved patient engagement, and lower no-show rates.

Challenges of Virtual Assistants

Despite their promise, adoption faces hurdles:

- **Accuracy**: Incorrect advice or misunderstood input can be harmful.
- **Privacy concerns**: Conversations often involve sensitive health data that must be secured.
- **Integration**: Virtual assistants must work smoothly with EHRs, scheduling systems, and hospital workflows.
- **Trust and acceptance**: Both clinicians and patients may be skeptical of AI advice, especially in critical cases.

Takeaway

Virtual assistants are changing the way clinicians and patients interact with healthcare. For doctors, they reduce administrative burdens and provide instant access to critical information. For patients, they offer continuous guidance, reminders, and education beyond the clinic walls. While issues of accuracy, privacy, and trust must be managed, virtual assistants represent a powerful step toward more connected, efficient, and patient-centered healthcare.

Reducing Burnout and Improving Workflow Efficiency

Clinician burnout is one of the most serious issues in modern healthcare. Long hours, overwhelming administrative tasks, and the constant demand for accuracy take a heavy toll on doctors, nurses, and other staff. Burnout not only affects providers' well-being but also reduces quality of care and increases medical errors. AI offers tools to reduce this burden by streamlining workflows, cutting paperwork, and restoring focus on patients.

The Reality of Burnout

Studies show that more than **40% of physicians** report symptoms of burnout, such as exhaustion, depersonalization, and reduced sense of accomplishment. Key contributors include:

- **Administrative overload**: endless charting, billing, and reporting.
- **Inefficient workflows**: time wasted searching through fragmented electronic health records.
- **High patient loads**: not enough time per visit.
- **Work–life imbalance**: long shifts with little recovery time.

Without intervention, burnout leads to higher staff turnover, shortages of specialists, and decreased patient satisfaction.

How AI Improves Workflow Efficiency

AI systems reduce burnout by **taking on repetitive, time-consuming tasks** and improving workflow design. Key contributions include:

- **Automated documentation**: Voice recognition and NLP-powered scribes convert conversations into structured notes, cutting documentation time by up to 70%.
- **Smart EHR navigation**: AI tools summarize patient records and highlight key changes, reducing time wasted clicking through pages.
- **Optimized scheduling**: Predictive scheduling balances workloads, preventing clinicians from being overloaded while minimizing patient wait times.
- **Decision support**: AI suggests relevant diagnoses, treatment guidelines, and medication checks, reducing mental strain from information overload.
- **Task delegation**: Virtual assistants handle reminders, routine queries, and follow-up communication.

The result: clinicians spend more time with patients and less time with screens.

Real-World Results

Hospitals and clinics adopting AI-powered workflow tools report:

- **Increased efficiency**: Some physicians save 1–2 hours per day on paperwork.
- **Reduced stress**: Staff feel less overwhelmed by administrative demands.
- **Better patient engagement**: More time for meaningful conversations improves trust and care quality.
- **Lower turnover**: Staff retention improves when work feels manageable and rewarding.

For example, AI scribes such as **Nuance DAX** are being used in U.S. hospitals to automate note-taking, cutting burnout rates and significantly boosting clinician satisfaction.

Balancing AI and Human Roles

AI can improve workflows, but it cannot solve burnout alone. Technology must be implemented carefully:

- If poorly designed, AI tools may **add complexity** rather than reduce it.
- Staff need training to integrate AI seamlessly into daily practice.
- Emotional stress from patient care still requires broader support systems, such as counseling and better work–life balance policies.

Takeaway

Burnout in healthcare is a crisis that threatens both providers and patients. AI helps by removing unnecessary burdens, optimizing workflows, and freeing clinicians to focus on what matters most: caring for people. When combined with supportive workplace practices, AI has the potential to not only improve efficiency but also restore meaning and balance to healthcare work.

CHAPTER 5

AI in Drug Discovery and Research

Accelerating Pharmaceutical R&D with AI Models

Developing a new drug is one of the most expensive and time-consuming processes in healthcare. On average, it takes **10–15 years** and costs billions of dollars to bring a single drug from concept to market. Many potential drugs fail during trials, wasting years of work and resources. AI is changing this landscape by accelerating research, reducing costs, and increasing the chances of success.

The Traditional Bottlenecks in Drug Development

Drug discovery follows a complex path:

1. **Target identification** – finding the biological process or protein linked to a disease.
2. **Compound screening** – testing thousands of molecules for potential activity.
3. **Preclinical testing** – evaluating safety in cells and animal models.
4. **Clinical trials** – proving safety and effectiveness in humans.

The process is slow because:

- Screening millions of compounds in labs is time-consuming.
- Human-driven analysis of biological pathways is limited.
- High failure rates in clinical trials delay progress.

How AI Speeds Up R&D

AI tackles these bottlenecks by analyzing massive datasets far faster than humans. Models trained on biological, chemical, and clinical data can:

- **Predict drug–target interactions**: AI identifies which molecules are most likely to bind to a disease-related protein.

- **Screen compounds virtually**: Instead of physically testing millions of molecules, AI narrows down the most promising candidates.
- **Repurpose existing drugs**: Algorithms find new uses for drugs already approved, cutting years off development time.
- **Optimize clinical trials**: AI helps design trials, select participants, and predict outcomes, reducing costly failures.

For example, instead of testing 1 million molecules in the lab, AI might identify 1,000 top candidates with the highest probability of success—saving years of work.

Real-World Success Stories

- **Insilico Medicine** used AI to design a novel drug for pulmonary fibrosis in less than 18 months, a process that typically takes several years.
- **Atomwise** applies AI to analyze billions of chemical compounds virtually, identifying promising treatments for diseases such as Ebola and multiple sclerosis.
- During **COVID-19**, AI models helped identify existing drugs that could be repurposed for managing the virus, accelerating treatment options when speed was critical.

These examples show that AI is not just theoretical—it is already reshaping pharmaceutical pipelines.

AI Beyond Molecules: Systems-Level Insights

AI does more than find drug candidates. It also uncovers **systems-level insights**:

- Identifying **biomarkers** that predict how patients will respond to drugs.
- Detecting potential **side effects** early by analyzing diverse datasets.
- Suggesting **drug combinations** that work better together than alone.

This broadens the scope of research from single molecules to whole patient populations.

Challenges Ahead

Despite the promise, integrating AI into pharmaceutical R&D faces obstacles:

- **Data quality**: Incomplete or biased datasets can lead to false predictions.
- **Validation**: AI-generated candidates still require lab and clinical testing.
- **Trust**: Researchers must understand how AI models reach conclusions, especially when lives are at stake.
- **Regulation**: Drug approvals involve strict oversight, and regulators must adapt to AI-driven processes.

Takeaway

AI models are accelerating pharmaceutical research by predicting drug interactions, screening compounds virtually, and even repurposing existing drugs. What once took a decade can now be achieved in a fraction of the time. While challenges of trust, data quality, and regulation remain, AI is rapidly becoming a cornerstone of drug discovery—reshaping the timeline of innovation and bringing treatments to patients faster than ever before.

Drug Repurposing and Molecular Simulations

Developing a brand-new drug from scratch is slow and costly, but what if existing drugs could be given new life? This is the promise of **drug repurposing**, where medications already approved for one condition are tested for effectiveness against another. Combined with **molecular simulations powered by AI**, this approach is accelerating discovery, lowering costs, and bringing treatments to patients much faster.

The Case for Drug Repurposing

Traditional drug development faces high failure rates in clinical trials. Repurposing offers a shortcut:

- **Safety is already proven** since the drug has been tested in humans.
- **Regulatory approval is faster** because much of the groundwork is complete.
- **Costs are lower** compared to inventing a new molecule.

Classic examples include:

- **Aspirin**, originally developed as a painkiller, now widely used to prevent heart attacks and strokes.
- **Thalidomide**, once infamous for birth defects, later repurposed to treat multiple myeloma.
- During the **COVID-19 pandemic**, drugs like remdesivir and dexamethasone were repurposed quickly to manage severe infections.

AI makes this process more systematic by scanning massive databases of drug properties, patient data, and molecular interactions.

How AI Enhances Repurposing

AI algorithms can uncover hidden links between drugs and diseases by:

- **Analyzing molecular structures** to predict how an existing drug might interact with new targets.

- **Mining clinical data** to detect patterns—such as patients taking a drug for one condition showing unexpected improvements in another.
- **Predicting side effects** early by comparing chemical properties across multiple drugs.

This enables scientists to prioritize the most promising candidates for lab and clinical testing.

Molecular Simulations with AI

Molecular simulations are another area where AI accelerates discovery. Traditionally, simulating how a molecule binds to a protein (known as **molecular docking**) requires vast computing power and time. AI-driven simulations streamline this process by:

- **Predicting 3D interactions** between drugs and proteins with high accuracy.
- **Exploring millions of variations** of molecules virtually, without needing to synthesize them all.
- **Identifying binding hotspots** where drugs can most effectively attach to disease-related proteins.

For instance, AI systems can model how a potential drug might block a viral protein—such as the spike protein in coronaviruses—helping researchers design treatments faster.

Real-World Applications

- **AlphaFold**, developed by DeepMind, revolutionized biology by predicting protein structures with near-laboratory accuracy. This breakthrough is already fueling drug discovery by giving researchers detailed maps of previously unknown protein shapes.
- **BenevolentAI** used AI-driven molecular analysis to identify baricitinib, an arthritis drug, as a treatment option for COVID-19—repurposed in record time.

- **Simulation platforms** like Schrödinger use AI to design and test molecules virtually, reducing trial-and-error in the lab.

Challenges and Limitations

While powerful, drug repurposing and molecular simulations face hurdles:

- **False leads**: Not every AI-predicted match works in the real world.
- **Complex biology**: Diseases often involve multiple pathways that simple models may overlook.
- **Data quality**: Biased or incomplete datasets can misguide predictions.
- **Regulatory adaptation**: Agencies are still adapting rules for AI-driven repurposing.

Takeaway

AI-powered drug repurposing and molecular simulations are reshaping how treatments are discovered. By analyzing existing drugs and virtually testing molecular interactions, researchers can bypass years of lab work, cut costs, and deliver therapies faster. While challenges of accuracy and regulation remain, these tools mark a new era where old drugs find new purpose, and new drugs can be designed with unprecedented speed.

Clinical Trial Optimization and Patient Recruitment

Even after a promising drug is discovered, one of the biggest hurdles is proving its safety and effectiveness in humans. This happens through **clinical trials**, which are notoriously slow, expensive, and often unsuccessful. Nearly **80–90% of drugs** entering trials never make it to approval. AI is transforming this process by making trials more efficient, improving patient recruitment, and increasing the chances of success.

The Bottlenecks in Clinical Trials

Running a clinical trial is like managing a small city of science and logistics:

- **Recruitment struggles**: Finding enough qualified patients who meet eligibility criteria can take years.
- **High dropout rates**: Patients may leave due to side effects, long travel, or poor communication.
- **Data management challenges**: Trials generate massive datasets, from lab results to wearable monitoring.
- **Cost and time**: Average costs for a single trial can exceed hundreds of millions of dollars.

These barriers delay access to life-saving treatments and drive up drug prices.

How AI Improves Patient Recruitment

Recruiting the right patients is critical to success, and AI makes this faster and more precise:

- **EHR mining**: AI scans electronic health records to identify patients who meet trial criteria.
- **Genomic matching**: For precision medicine, AI can find patients whose genetic profiles fit the trial requirements.
- **Predictive outreach**: Algorithms predict which patients are most likely to participate and stay engaged, improving retention.
- **Diversity optimization**: AI ensures recruitment includes patients across age groups, ethnicities, and regions, addressing long-standing bias in clinical research.

For example, a cancer trial can use AI to scan thousands of hospital records and flag patients with the right tumor mutations, cutting recruitment time from years to months.

AI in Trial Design and Monitoring

Beyond recruitment, AI helps optimize trial operations:

- **Adaptive trial design**: AI suggests modifications (e.g., dosage adjustments) as data emerges, keeping studies relevant.
- **Site selection**: Algorithms identify hospitals or regions with the highest concentration of eligible patients, reducing logistical challenges.
- **Real-time monitoring**: Wearables and connected devices feed continuous data, allowing researchers to track side effects or treatment responses more accurately.
- **Predicting dropout risk**: AI flags patients likely to withdraw, enabling intervention before it happens.

These innovations make trials leaner, smarter, and more patient-friendly.

Real-World Examples

- **Deep 6 AI** uses natural language processing to search unstructured clinical notes, matching patients to trials in minutes rather than months.
- **Pfizer and Novartis** have used AI-driven recruitment platforms to accelerate oncology trials, improving diversity and efficiency.
- During the **COVID-19 pandemic**, AI helped rapidly identify trial participants worldwide, speeding vaccine development.

Challenges and Cautions

While AI is powerful, clinical trials face unique challenges:

- **Data privacy**: Recruiting from medical records requires strict consent and compliance with regulations like HIPAA and GDPR.
- **Bias**: If AI systems rely on biased datasets, recruitment may still exclude underserved populations.
- **Regulatory adaptation**: Authorities are cautious about approving AI-assisted designs, requiring rigorous validation.
- **Human oversight**: Final decisions must still involve doctors and researchers to ensure patient safety.

Takeaway

AI is streamlining one of the hardest parts of drug development: clinical trials. By improving patient recruitment, optimizing trial design, and enabling real-time monitoring, AI reduces costs, accelerates timelines, and increases trial success rates. While challenges remain in privacy, bias, and regulation, AI-powered clinical trials are already proving their value in bringing new treatments to patients faster.

Predictive Models for Treatment Efficacy

One of the hardest questions in medicine is: *Will this treatment work for this patient?* Traditional approaches rely on population averages from clinical trials, but individual patients often respond very differently. AI-powered predictive models are changing this by analyzing multiple data sources to estimate the likelihood that a specific treatment will succeed for a specific patient. This reduces trial-and-error medicine, improves outcomes, and lowers costs.

Why Predictive Models Matter

Treatment decisions often involve uncertainty:

- A cancer drug may work for some patients but fail for others with the same diagnosis.
- Side effects can vary widely depending on genetics, age, or coexisting conditions.
- Doctors must balance risks and benefits without knowing exactly how each patient will respond.

Predictive models bring clarity by using patient data to forecast treatment efficacy and safety in advance.

How AI Builds Predictive Models

AI predictive models are trained on vast datasets, including:

- **Genomic profiles** to identify genetic mutations influencing drug response.
- **Electronic health records (EHRs)** with treatment histories and outcomes.
- **Imaging and pathology data** to link biological patterns with therapy effectiveness.
- **Wearable and real-time monitoring data** to assess lifestyle and physiological factors.

By combining these sources, AI creates a personalized prediction—answering questions like:

- "What's the likelihood this chemotherapy will shrink the tumor?"
- "How well will this diabetes medication control blood sugar for this patient?"
- "Is this patient at high risk of adverse effects from the proposed treatment?"

Real-World Applications

1. Oncology
AI models analyze tumor genomics and prior treatment responses to predict which cancer therapies—chemotherapy, immunotherapy, or targeted drugs—are most likely to work. For example, AI has been used to identify melanoma patients who will respond best to immune checkpoint inhibitors.

2. Cardiology
Predictive tools estimate how patients with heart failure will respond to different drug regimens, guiding personalized treatment choices and reducing hospital readmissions.

3. Psychiatry
AI models analyze speech, behavior, and genetics to predict which antidepressants are most likely to work for a given patient, reducing the frustrating trial-and-error approach common in mental health care.

4. Chronic Disease Management
AI predicts which patients will benefit most from lifestyle interventions versus medication for conditions like diabetes or hypertension.

Benefits of Predictive Treatment Models

- **Personalized therapy**: Care is tailored to the individual, not the average.
- **Fewer side effects**: Patients avoid ineffective or harmful treatments.
- **Faster results**: Doctors can skip failed first-line therapies and go directly to the most promising option.
- **Cost efficiency**: Resources are focused on treatments with the highest likelihood of success.

Challenges and Limitations

- **Data quality**: Incomplete or biased data can weaken predictions.
- **Transparency**: Many AI models function as "black boxes," making it hard to explain why a treatment is predicted to work.
- **Validation**: Predictive accuracy must be proven across diverse populations.
- **Ethics**: If AI predicts poor efficacy, should a treatment still be offered to give patients hope?

Takeaway

Predictive models for treatment efficacy mark a shift toward true precision medicine. By forecasting how well a therapy will work for each patient, AI reduces trial-and-error, improves outcomes, and saves time and money. While transparency, validation, and ethics must be addressed, these models are already proving that the future of medicine is not just about finding new drugs—it's about making sure the right patient gets the right treatment at the right time.

CHAPTER 6

Robotics and Smart Devices in Healthcare

Surgical Robots: Precision and Minimally Invasive Procedures

Surgery has always been one of the most demanding fields in medicine, requiring extreme precision, steady hands, and years of training. Even small errors can have life-threatening consequences. In recent years, **surgical robots** have entered the operating room, transforming what surgeons can achieve. These systems, guided by human expertise and enhanced by AI, allow for procedures that are more precise, less invasive, and safer for patients.

The Rise of Surgical Robotics

The most widely known system is the **da Vinci Surgical System**, introduced in the early 2000s. It allows surgeons to perform complex operations through tiny incisions using robotic arms controlled from a console. Instead of large cuts, the surgeon manipulates miniature tools with millimeter-level accuracy.

What started in urology and gynecology has now expanded into cardiac, orthopedic, and general surgery. Surgical robotics is no longer experimental—it is becoming standard in many hospitals worldwide.

Why Robots in Surgery?

Robotic systems address some of the biggest challenges in traditional surgery:

- **Enhanced precision**: Robots eliminate hand tremors and allow for movements smaller than a millimeter.
- **Better visualization**: High-definition 3D cameras give surgeons magnified views of tissue structures.
- **Minimally invasive access**: Procedures that once required large incisions can now be done with small keyhole cuts.

- **Reduced fatigue**: Surgeons can operate from an ergonomic console, decreasing physical strain during long procedures.

The result is surgery that is both safer for patients and more sustainable for surgeons.

Benefits for Patients

Minimally invasive robotic surgery translates into clear advantages for patients:

- **Smaller incisions** → less pain and scarring.
- **Lower risk of infection** due to reduced tissue exposure.
- **Shorter hospital stays** and faster recovery times.
- **Higher precision** → fewer complications and improved outcomes.

For example, in prostate surgery, robotic assistance allows for greater precision in nerve-sparing techniques, preserving urinary and sexual function more effectively than traditional approaches.

AI and the Future of Surgical Robotics

Today's surgical robots are primarily tools guided by human surgeons. But with AI integration, they are becoming more intelligent:

- **Automated assistance**: AI can stabilize instruments or guide the surgeon to the exact location of interest.
- **Skill enhancement**: Systems analyze past procedures, offering suggestions or highlighting anatomical structures in real time.
- **Training support**: Robots with AI feedback help train new surgeons by scoring performance and providing corrections.
- **Partial automation**: For routine steps (like suturing), AI may perform tasks under supervision, speeding up procedures.

This doesn't mean replacing surgeons—it means giving them smarter tools to extend their capabilities.

Challenges of Robotic Surgery

Despite the benefits, challenges remain:

- **High cost**: Robotic systems and maintenance are expensive, limiting availability in lower-resource hospitals.
- **Learning curve**: Surgeons need extensive training to use these systems effectively.
- **Access inequality**: Patients in rural or underfunded areas may not benefit from robotic advancements.
- **Reliability**: While rare, technical failures in surgery can be serious and require backup protocols.

Takeaway

Surgical robots are redefining what is possible in the operating room. By enhancing precision, enabling minimally invasive techniques, and reducing recovery times, they benefit both surgeons and patients. With AI integration, surgical robots will move from being sophisticated tools to intelligent partners, ensuring safer, faster, and more effective procedures. The future of surgery is not man versus machine—it is man and machine working together for better outcomes.

Smart Prosthetics and Rehabilitation Technologies

Losing a limb or recovering from a serious injury can be life-changing. Traditional prosthetics and rehabilitation methods help patients regain function, but they often have limitations. Today, advances in robotics, sensors, and AI are creating **smart prosthetics and rehabilitation technologies** that go far beyond simple replacements. These innovations restore mobility, enhance independence, and improve quality of life for millions of people worldwide.

From Mechanical to Smart Prosthetics

Older prosthetics were largely mechanical—designed to provide basic mobility but with limited adaptability. Modern smart prosthetics, however, use **AI-driven control systems and advanced sensors** to mimic natural movement more closely.

Features include:

- **Myoelectric sensors**: Electrodes detect signals from muscles in the residual limb, translating them into movement commands for the prosthetic.
- **AI-driven pattern recognition**: Algorithms learn how the user intends to move and adjust the prosthetic's response over time.
- **Adaptive joints**: Smart knees and ankles automatically adjust to walking speed, terrain, or incline.
- **Feedback loops**: Some devices provide sensory feedback, allowing users to "feel" pressure or texture, improving coordination.

This means a person with a smart prosthetic hand can not only grip objects but also adjust the strength of the grip automatically— something impossible with older devices.

Robotics in Rehabilitation

Rehabilitation after stroke, spinal cord injury, or orthopedic surgery often requires months of intensive therapy. AI-powered rehabilitation robotics are making this process more effective by:

- **Robotic exoskeletons**: Wearable devices that assist with walking, enabling patients with partial paralysis to regain mobility.

- **AI-guided therapy robots**: Machines that provide repetitive motion exercises for arms and legs, adjusting intensity based on patient progress.
- **Virtual reality integration**: Combining robotics with VR environments makes therapy engaging, motivating patients to stick with programs.

For example, stroke patients using robotic-assisted therapy often recover faster because the robot provides precise, repetitive motion training while tracking performance data in real time.

Benefits for Patients

Smart prosthetics and rehabilitation technologies improve outcomes in several ways:

- **Greater independence**: Patients can perform daily activities—walking, grasping, climbing stairs—with more confidence.
- **Personalization**: AI systems learn from the individual user's patterns, creating a customized rehabilitation path.
- **Faster recovery**: Robotic therapy provides more consistent and intensive practice than traditional methods.
- **Improved quality of life**: Beyond physical recovery, these technologies reduce frustration and boost emotional well-being.

Real-World Applications

- Companies like **Össur** and **Ottobock** are producing AI-driven prosthetic legs that adjust automatically to terrain.
- **Ekso Bionics** has developed robotic exoskeletons used in rehabilitation centers to help patients relearn walking.
- **ReWalk Robotics** provides wearable robotic suits approved for personal use, giving mobility to people with spinal cord injuries.

These are not futuristic concepts—they are already being used in clinics and, increasingly, in homes.

Challenges and Limitations

Despite progress, hurdles remain:

- **Cost**: Advanced prosthetics and exoskeletons are expensive and not always covered by insurance.
- **Accessibility**: Many technologies are available only in specialized rehabilitation centers.
- **Training**: Patients need time to adapt to new devices, which requires dedicated support.
- **Durability**: High-tech devices must withstand daily wear and tear, which can be challenging.

Takeaway

Smart prosthetics and rehabilitation technologies are transforming recovery and mobility. By combining robotics, sensors, and AI, they enable movements that feel more natural, support faster rehabilitation, and give patients greater independence. While cost and accessibility remain barriers, the direction is clear: the future of prosthetics and rehabilitation is not just functional—it is intelligent, adaptive, and life-enhancing.

AI in Elderly and Disability Care Robotics

As populations age worldwide, healthcare systems are under increasing pressure to care for elderly and disabled individuals. Many face daily challenges—mobility issues, chronic illnesses, or the need for continuous support. At the same time, shortages of caregivers and rising costs create significant gaps in care. **AI-powered robotics** is emerging as a vital solution, providing assistance, monitoring, and companionship that help people live more independently and safely.

Why Robotics in Elderly and Disability Care?

Traditional caregiving depends heavily on human support, which is not always available or affordable. AI-driven robots fill this gap by:

- Assisting with **physical tasks**, such as lifting, walking support, or mobility aid.
- Providing **daily reminders** for medications, hydration, or appointments.
- Monitoring health indicators to detect risks early.
- Offering **companionship**, reducing loneliness and social isolation.

The goal is not to replace caregivers but to extend their reach and improve quality of life for those who need continuous support.

Types of Care Robots

1. **Mobility and Assistance Robots**
   - Exoskeletons and robotic walkers help elderly or disabled patients move safely.
   - AI adjusts support based on the person's stability, pace, and environment.
2. **Health Monitoring Robots**
   - Robots with sensors track vital signs, detect falls, and send alerts to caregivers.
   - Some are integrated with wearable devices to provide continuous updates.
3. **Social Companion Robots**
   - Devices like **Paro**, a therapeutic robot seal, or **ElliQ**, an AI-powered companion, provide emotional support.
   - They engage in conversation, play music, or encourage cognitive exercises.
4. **Household Assistance Robots**
   - Robots that help with daily tasks—fetching items, reminding about chores, or guiding patients around the house.

Real-World Applications

- **Toyota's Human Support Robot (HSR)** helps people with disabilities by picking up objects, opening doors, or assisting with daily activities.
- **Pepper**, a humanoid robot, has been tested in elderly care homes to provide companionship and support group activities.
- **Care-o-bot** systems in Europe are designed to assist with household tasks and provide interaction.
- Fall-detection robots integrated with AI vision systems are being used in nursing homes to prevent injuries.

These technologies are already demonstrating measurable benefits, such as reduced falls, better medication adherence, and improved emotional well-being.

Benefits for Patients and Caregivers

- **Increased independence**: Elderly and disabled individuals can perform more tasks without constant supervision.
- **Safety**: AI-powered monitoring reduces risks of falls, missed medications, or unnoticed health deterioration.
- **Relief for caregivers**: Robots handle routine tasks, allowing human caregivers to focus on emotional and complex care.
- **Social engagement**: Companion robots help reduce loneliness, a major contributor to poor health outcomes among the elderly.

Challenges and Limitations

Despite progress, adoption faces barriers:

- **Cost and accessibility**: Advanced robots remain expensive and out of reach for many households.
- **Trust and acceptance**: Some elderly patients may feel uncomfortable with machines replacing human interaction.

- **Technical limitations**: Robots still struggle with complex, unpredictable environments.
- **Ethical concerns**: Over-reliance on machines may risk reducing human-to-human contact in care.

Takeaway

AI-driven robotics is transforming elderly and disability care by offering mobility support, monitoring health, assisting with daily tasks, and even providing companionship. These tools cannot replace the empathy of human caregivers, but they extend care capacity, improve safety, and enhance independence. In the face of aging populations and caregiver shortages, care robotics may become not just a convenience but a necessity.

The Rise of Hospital Automation and Delivery Robots

Hospitals are complex ecosystems. Beyond treating patients, they must manage an enormous flow of supplies—medications, linens, meals, lab samples, and equipment. Traditionally, these tasks rely on human staff, but in busy hospitals, this work is time-consuming and inefficient. **AI-powered delivery and automation robots** are stepping in to take over these routine tasks, allowing healthcare workers to focus more on direct patient care.

Why Hospitals Need Automation

Healthcare staff are often overwhelmed, and much of their time is spent on non-clinical tasks. Nurses, for example, may spend hours transporting medications, retrieving supplies, or delivering lab samples instead of being at the bedside.

These inefficiencies lead to:

- Longer patient wait times.
- Staff fatigue and burnout.
- Increased operational costs.

By automating logistics and routine services, hospitals can run more efficiently while improving staff satisfaction.

Delivery Robots in Action

Delivery robots are already working in hospitals worldwide. They can:

- **Transport medications** securely from the pharmacy to patient units.
- **Deliver meals, linens, or medical supplies** across different departments.
- **Carry lab samples** to testing facilities quickly and safely.
- **Navigate autonomously** using AI-based mapping and obstacle detection, even in crowded hallways.

For example, robots like **Aethon's TUG** can carry hundreds of pounds of supplies and navigate elevators to deliver items directly to nursing stations.

Hospital Automation Beyond Delivery

AI-driven automation extends beyond delivery robots:

- **Automated disinfection robots** use UV light to sanitize rooms, reducing infection risks.
- **Inventory management systems** powered by AI track supplies and predict when reorders are needed.
- **Automated guided vehicles (AGVs)** transport waste or biohazard materials safely.

- **Pharmacy automation** uses robotic systems to prepare, package, and dispense medications with high accuracy.

These innovations reduce human error and create safer, more reliable hospital operations.

Benefits for Hospitals and Patients

Hospital automation delivers value on multiple levels:

- **For staff**: Less time on routine logistics, more time for patient care.
- **For patients**: Faster services, reduced infection risks, and smoother hospital experiences.
- **For hospitals**: Lower labor costs, improved efficiency, and fewer supply chain bottlenecks.

In some hospitals, introducing delivery robots has reduced nurse time spent on logistics by up to **20–30%**, directly increasing time available for patient care.

Challenges and Considerations

Despite the promise, hospital automation faces hurdles:

- **High upfront costs** for robots and infrastructure.
- **Integration issues** with existing hospital layouts and IT systems.
- **Maintenance needs** to ensure robots remain reliable.
- **Acceptance** by staff, who may worry about robots replacing human jobs rather than supporting them.

Takeaway

Hospital automation and delivery robots are reshaping the way healthcare facilities operate. By handling logistics, sanitation, and routine tasks, robots free healthcare professionals to focus on what matters most—treating patients. While cost and integration challenges remain, the rise of hospital automation signals a future where healthcare systems are not only smarter but also more human-centered, as staff are relieved from routine burdens and patients benefit from faster, safer, and more efficient care.

CHAPTER 7

Ethical, Legal, and Security Challenges

Patient Privacy and HIPAA/GDPR Compliance

AI in healthcare depends on data—electronic health records, imaging, genomics, and even data from wearable devices. While this information powers better diagnosis and treatment, it also raises serious questions: *Who owns patient data? How is it protected? What happens if it is misused?* Ensuring privacy and compliance with regulations like **HIPAA** (Health Insurance Portability and Accountability Act in the U.S.) and **GDPR** (General Data Protection Regulation in Europe) is essential for building trust in AI-driven healthcare.

Why Privacy Matters in Healthcare AI

Medical data is among the most sensitive information a person has. A breach can lead not only to identity theft but also to stigma, discrimination, or misuse by insurers and employers. As AI requires massive datasets, privacy challenges intensify:

- **Scale of data**: Millions of records may be needed to train AI models.
- **Diversity of sources**: Data comes from hospitals, labs, insurers, and consumer devices.
- **Potential misuse**: Without safeguards, data could be sold or exploited for non-medical purposes.

Protecting privacy is not just a legal obligation—it is a moral foundation of patient trust.

HIPAA: The U.S. Standard

HIPAA, enacted in 1996, governs the use, storage, and sharing of health information in the United States. Under HIPAA:

- **Protected Health Information (PHI)** includes any identifiable medical data.
- Organizations must ensure **data security** (encryption, access control, audit trails).
- Patients have rights to access and request corrections to their data.
- Sharing data requires **consent**, except in certain cases like public health emergencies.

For AI developers, HIPAA compliance means strict controls on how health data is accessed and anonymized.

GDPR: The European Framework

The GDPR, implemented in 2018, is one of the strictest privacy laws in the world. While broader than healthcare, it applies directly to medical data. GDPR emphasizes:

- **Consent**: Patients must explicitly agree to how their data is collected and used.
- **Right to be forgotten**: Patients can demand that their data be erased.
- **Transparency**: Organizations must clearly explain how data is processed.
- **Accountability**: Heavy fines can be imposed for violations.

For AI, GDPR sets higher standards: not just protecting data but also ensuring patients understand how their information fuels algorithms.

AI-Specific Privacy Challenges

AI creates unique pressures on privacy laws:

- **De-identification limits**: Even anonymized data can sometimes be re-identified with advanced analytics.
- **Cross-border data use**: Global research often requires data sharing across countries with different regulations.
- **Continuous monitoring**: Wearables and home devices generate constant streams of sensitive health data.
- **Black-box models**: When AI decisions are opaque, patients may worry about how their data is actually being used.

Strategies for Secure AI in Healthcare

To balance innovation with privacy, healthcare organizations and AI developers are adopting safeguards such as:

- **Data anonymization and pseudonymization**: Removing or masking identifiers before analysis.
- **Federated learning**: Training AI models on decentralized data (e.g., in hospitals) without moving the raw data.
- **Encryption and secure storage**: Ensuring data cannot be accessed or altered by unauthorized users.
- **Audit trails**: Tracking every data access and AI decision for accountability.
- **Explainability tools**: Showing patients how their data contributes to AI-driven insights.

Takeaway

Patient privacy is the foundation of ethical AI in healthcare. Regulations like HIPAA and GDPR set important guardrails, but the rise of AI introduces new risks that require stronger safeguards. Building trust means going beyond compliance—using technologies like federated learning, robust encryption, and transparent consent to ensure patients' most personal data remains protected. Without privacy, AI cannot succeed in healthcare; with it, patients and providers can embrace innovation with confidence.

Bias and Fairness in Medical AI Algorithms

AI in healthcare promises faster diagnoses, personalized treatments, and better outcomes. But these benefits are only possible if the technology works equally well for everyone. Unfortunately, medical AI systems are vulnerable to **bias**, meaning they may perform better for some groups of patients than others. Bias in healthcare is not new, but when encoded into AI algorithms, it risks amplifying existing inequalities at scale. Ensuring fairness is one of the greatest ethical challenges in AI adoption.

Where Bias Comes From

Bias in medical AI often originates from the data used to train algorithms. Common sources include:

- **Unbalanced datasets**: If most training data comes from one demographic (e.g., white male patients), the model may not perform well for women or minorities.
- **Historical inequities**: Healthcare systems have long documented disparities in access and treatment; AI trained on this history may learn and replicate the same patterns.

- **Proxy variables**: AI sometimes relies on indirect signals, such as income level or ZIP code, which may reflect socioeconomic status rather than actual health risks.
- **Device bias**: Medical devices, like pulse oximeters, have been shown to be less accurate for darker skin tones, and AI trained on such data inherits those flaws.

Real-World Examples of Bias

Bias is not theoretical—it has already been observed in healthcare AI:

- A widely used U.S. algorithm for predicting which patients need extra care was found to **systematically underestimate the needs of Black patients**, because it used healthcare spending as a proxy for illness, ignoring structural inequities in access.
- AI dermatology tools trained mostly on images of light skin performed poorly when identifying skin cancers on darker skin.
- Natural language processing systems trained on clinician notes sometimes picked up biased language, influencing how patient risk was scored.

These examples show how easily AI can perpetuate or even worsen disparities.

Why Fairness Matters

Biased algorithms don't just create statistical errors—they can cause real harm:

- **Delayed diagnosis** for underrepresented groups.
- **Inequitable access** to treatments or preventive care.
- **Loss of trust** in healthcare technology, especially in already marginalized communities.

Fairness in AI is not just a technical issue—it is a matter of justice and patient safety.

Strategies to Reduce Bias

Researchers, hospitals, and regulators are working on ways to ensure fairness in medical AI:

- **Diverse datasets**: Including data from varied ethnicities, ages, genders, and socioeconomic groups.
- **Bias audits**: Regularly testing models to check for unequal performance across subgroups.
- **Explainable AI (XAI)**: Making models transparent so biases can be identified and corrected.
- **Algorithmic fairness techniques**: Adjusting models during training to balance predictions across groups.
- **Human oversight**: Ensuring AI supports—not replaces—clinicians' judgment, with doctors aware of potential biases.

Regulatory and Ethical Considerations

Under **GDPR in Europe**, patients have a "right to explanation" when AI makes healthcare decisions, which forces organizations to examine fairness. In the U.S., regulators are beginning to require evidence that AI tools perform equally well across populations before approval. Ethical guidelines stress that fairness must be monitored continuously, not just at the point of development.

Takeaway

Bias in medical AI is not just a technical flaw—it is a moral and clinical risk. Algorithms that work well only for some patients undermine the promise of AI-driven healthcare. By ensuring diverse data, conducting fairness audits, and maintaining human oversight, healthcare systems can build AI that serves everyone equally. Fairness is not optional; it is the foundation of ethical, trustworthy AI in medicine.

Liability and Accountability in AI-Based Decisions

AI in healthcare is moving from research labs into real-world clinics, where it influences diagnoses, treatment choices, and even surgical procedures. But as AI takes on greater responsibility, a critical question arises: *Who is accountable when something goes wrong?* In medicine, errors can mean delayed diagnoses, harmful treatments, or even death. Unlike traditional tools, AI decisions may be opaque, raising complex legal and ethical debates about liability.

The Traditional Standard of Accountability

In healthcare, accountability has historically been clear:

- **Physicians** are responsible for clinical decisions.
- **Hospitals** are responsible for maintaining safe systems.
- **Manufacturers** are accountable for faulty devices or drugs.

When AI enters the picture, these lines blur. If an AI system suggests a treatment and a doctor follows it, who bears responsibility if the outcome is harmful—the doctor, the hospital, or the AI developer?

Scenarios of AI-Related Liability

1. **AI as a Support Tool**
   - If AI provides recommendations but the doctor makes the final decision, liability largely remains with the physician.
   - However, if the AI's advice was misleading due to poor design, the developer could also share responsibility.
2. **AI as a Semi-Autonomous System**
   - In robotic surgery, if a robotic arm makes a technical error, liability may fall on both the surgeon supervising the procedure and the manufacturer.

3. **AI as a Fully Autonomous Actor**
   o As AI moves toward autonomous diagnosis or treatment selection, accountability becomes more complex. If there is no direct human decision, assigning liability is far less straightforward.

Legal Gaps in Current Frameworks

Existing laws were not designed for AI-driven healthcare. Challenges include:

- **Opacity of algorithms**: Black-box models make it hard to explain why a decision was made. Without transparency, proving negligence is difficult.
- **Shared responsibility**: Multiple stakeholders—clinicians, hospitals, software vendors—may all be partly responsible.
- **Cross-border regulation**: AI tools may be developed in one country, deployed in another, and used on international patient populations. Legal accountability is unclear in these cases.

Emerging Approaches

Governments and regulators are exploring ways to manage liability:

- **Strict liability for manufacturers**: Holding developers accountable if their AI system malfunctions, similar to how defective medical devices are regulated.
- **Shared liability models**: Dividing accountability between clinicians, hospitals, and AI vendors depending on the context.
- **Algorithm certification**: Requiring AI tools to undergo rigorous testing before approval, with clear standards for performance and safety.
- **Audit and traceability requirements**: Ensuring AI decisions are logged and traceable so that accountability can be assigned if harm occurs.

Ethical Considerations

Beyond legal frameworks, accountability has ethical dimensions:

- **Trust in AI**: Patients must know that if AI harms them, someone is responsible.
- **Duty of care**: Physicians should not blindly follow AI recommendations but use them as one input among many.
- **Transparency**: Patients deserve to know when AI is involved in their care and how decisions are made.

Takeaway

AI complicates the question of accountability in medicine. While doctors, hospitals, and manufacturers have clear responsibilities in traditional healthcare, AI creates gray areas where liability is shared. Building trust requires both legal reforms and ethical safeguards—ensuring that patients are protected, errors are addressed, and AI is deployed responsibly. In the end, AI may assist in decisions, but accountability must always remain human-centered.

Cybersecurity Threats in AI Healthcare Systems

As healthcare becomes increasingly digital, hospitals, clinics, and research centers are relying on AI to store, analyze, and process sensitive data. But this integration also makes healthcare one of the most attractive targets for cybercriminals. From ransomware attacks on hospitals to theft of patient records, cybersecurity threats in AI-powered systems pose serious risks to patient safety and trust.

Why Healthcare Is a Prime Target

Healthcare data is extremely valuable on the black market. Unlike credit cards, which can be canceled, medical records contain permanent information—diagnoses, Social Security numbers, addresses, and even genomic data. Criminals use this information for identity theft, insurance fraud, or blackmail.

AI systems make healthcare even more vulnerable because they:

- Rely on **large, centralized datasets** that hackers can target.
- Often connect across multiple systems (EHRs, imaging, labs, wearables), increasing attack surfaces.
- Use algorithms that, if manipulated, can lead to **incorrect diagnoses or treatment recommendations**.

Common Cybersecurity Threats

1. **Ransomware Attacks**
   - Hackers lock hospital systems and demand payment to restore access. In 2020, such attacks forced hospitals in the U.S. and Europe to cancel surgeries and delay care.
2. **Data Breaches**
   - Theft of patient records is the most common attack. Breaches not only expose sensitive information but also erode trust in AI systems.
3. **Adversarial Attacks on AI Models**
   - By altering just a few pixels in a medical image, hackers can trick an AI system into misclassifying a scan (e.g., missing a tumor). This poses direct risks to patient safety.
4. **IoT and Device Vulnerabilities**
   - Wearables, infusion pumps, and smart medical devices connected to hospital networks can be hacked, allowing attackers to disrupt patient monitoring or drug delivery.
5. **Insider Threats**
   - Employees with access to systems may leak or misuse patient data, whether intentionally or accidentally.

Real-World Incidents

- In 2017, the **WannaCry ransomware attack** disrupted healthcare systems worldwide, particularly in the UK's National Health Service (NHS), causing mass cancellations of appointments and surgeries.
- Studies have shown that AI imaging models can be **fooled by adversarial attacks**, raising concerns about clinical deployment without proper safeguards.
- Several U.S. hospitals in recent years have faced **data breaches** exposing millions of patient records, often through weakly protected systems.

Securing AI in Healthcare

Protecting AI systems requires more than traditional cybersecurity—it demands specialized strategies tailored to healthcare:

- **Encryption**: Ensuring all data, at rest and in transit, is encrypted.
- **Zero-trust architecture**: Limiting system access strictly to verified users.
- **Federated learning**: Allowing AI models to train on decentralized hospital data without moving patient records into a central database.
- **Adversarial defense techniques**: Training AI to recognize and resist malicious input manipulations.
- **Continuous monitoring**: Using AI-driven cybersecurity tools to detect anomalies and stop attacks in real time.

Regulatory and Ethical Implications

HIPAA and GDPR already mandate strict protection of health data, but AI introduces new challenges.

Regulators are beginning to require:

- **Audit trails** of AI decisions.
- **Security certifications** for AI systems before deployment.
- **Transparency** around how patient data is stored and shared.

Ethically, hospitals must inform patients of potential risks and demonstrate that they are actively securing systems.

Takeaway

Cybersecurity threats in AI healthcare systems are not abstract—they are already disrupting hospitals and endangering patients. Protecting sensitive medical data and ensuring the integrity of AI models is just as important as medical accuracy itself. The future of AI in healthcare depends on building systems that are not only smart but also resilient against evolving cyberattacks. Trust, safety, and patient care cannot exist without security.

CHAPTER 8

The Future of AI in Healthcare

Emerging Trends: Digital Twins and Metaverse Medicine

The next frontier of AI in healthcare is not just smarter diagnostics or faster drug discovery—it is the creation of **digital worlds** that mirror and interact with real-life medicine. Two concepts leading this shift are **digital twins** and **metaverse medicine**. These emerging trends are pushing healthcare into spaces that, until recently, belonged only to science fiction.

What Are Digital Twins in Healthcare?

A **digital twin** is a virtual replica of a physical entity. In healthcare, it means creating a digital copy of a patient's body, organ, or even entire health system using AI, real-time data, and simulations.

For example:

- A **heart digital twin** can simulate blood flow and predict how it will respond to a new medication.
- A **whole-patient twin** integrates genetics, lifestyle, and medical history to forecast disease risk.
- At a **system level**, hospitals may use digital twins to model patient flow and resource needs.

Digital twins allow clinicians to test treatments virtually before applying them in real life, reducing trial-and-error and making care safer.

How AI Powers Digital Twins

AI enables digital twins by:

- **Analyzing patient data** from wearables, EHRs, and imaging.
- **Running simulations** that predict how the body will react to drugs, surgeries, or lifestyle changes.
- **Updating in real time** as new data is collected, ensuring the twin evolves with the patient.

This means a doctor could, for instance, simulate how a specific chemotherapy plan would affect an individual patient's tumor and organs, then adjust dosing for maximum benefit with minimal side effects.

Metaverse Medicine: Healthcare in Virtual Worlds

The **metaverse** is often associated with gaming or social media, but it also has serious implications for healthcare. With VR (virtual reality), AR (augmented reality), and AI, medicine is entering immersive digital environments that open up new possibilities:

- **Medical training**: Surgeons practice complex procedures in virtual operating rooms with AI-driven simulations.
- **Patient education**: Patients "walk through" their anatomy in VR to better understand their conditions and treatment options.
- **Telemedicine 2.0**: Virtual clinics in the metaverse let patients meet doctors in immersive spaces, improving engagement compared to video calls.
- **Mental health care**: VR therapy environments help patients manage phobias, PTSD, or anxiety in controlled digital settings.

In the future, patients may interact with digital replicas of themselves in the metaverse—seeing how lifestyle changes, therapies, or surgeries might affect their health outcomes.

Real-World Examples

- **Siemens Healthineers** is developing digital twin technology for cardiology, helping simulate heart behavior in different conditions.
- **Philips** has explored digital twins for personalized cancer treatment planning.
- **VR-based therapy programs** are already being used to treat PTSD in veterans by recreating safe but realistic exposure scenarios.
- Medical schools are adopting VR surgical training platforms, where AI-driven feedback helps students refine their skills.

Opportunities and Challenges

Opportunities:

- Hyper-personalized treatment based on simulations.
- Safer and faster training for healthcare professionals.
- Improved patient understanding and engagement.
- Virtual collaboration between global experts in shared digital environments.

Challenges:

- **Data complexity**: Building accurate digital twins requires massive, high-quality data streams.
- **Cost and infrastructure**: Advanced VR and simulation platforms are expensive.
- **Privacy**: Virtual replicas of patients raise new security concerns.
- **Accessibility**: Not all hospitals or patients will have equal access to these technologies.

Takeaway

Digital twins and metaverse medicine are pushing healthcare into a new era of simulation, personalization, and immersive care. By combining AI, real-time data, and virtual environments, they promise safer treatments, better training, and deeper patient engagement. While challenges of cost, privacy, and accessibility remain, these trends signal a future where healthcare is not limited to hospitals and clinics—but extended into intelligent, interactive digital worlds.

AI-Augmented Global Health and Telemedicine

Healthcare access remains deeply unequal across the globe. In many regions, shortages of doctors, limited infrastructure, and high costs prevent people from receiving timely care. AI and telemedicine are changing this picture by extending the reach of healthcare beyond physical hospitals and into homes, villages, and even smartphones. Together, they form a bridge between advanced medical knowledge and populations that have historically been underserved.

The Global Health Challenge

The World Health Organization (WHO) estimates a shortage of **10 million healthcare workers** worldwide by 2030, with the greatest gaps in low- and middle-income countries. Millions of people lack access to specialists such as radiologists, pathologists, or mental health professionals. Rural areas, refugee camps, and disaster zones often face the harshest shortages.

Without intervention, health disparities will continue to widen. AI-driven telemedicine offers a way to close this gap.

How AI Enhances Telemedicine

Telemedicine already allows patients to consult with doctors remotely via video calls or apps. AI strengthens this model by:

- **Symptom checkers and triage bots**: AI guides patients to the right level of care, reducing unnecessary ER visits.
- **Automated translation**: Real-time AI translation enables cross-language consultations, breaking down communication barriers.
- **Remote diagnostics**: AI algorithms analyze uploaded images (skin lesions, X-rays) and provide preliminary insights for doctors.
- **Monitoring at scale**: Wearables and mobile sensors track vital signs and transmit data for AI analysis, alerting clinicians only when intervention is needed.

This combination makes care more scalable, efficient, and personalized, even at a distance.

Real-World Examples

- In **India and Africa**, AI-powered telemedicine kiosks are being deployed in rural areas, offering automated vital sign checks, basic diagnostics, and links to remote doctors.
- **Babylon Health**, a UK-based platform, uses AI-driven symptom assessment combined with teleconsultations to serve millions of patients globally.
- During the **COVID-19 pandemic**, telemedicine supported by AI helped overwhelmed health systems triage patients, monitor recovery at home, and maintain continuity of care.

Benefits for Global Health

- **Increased access**: Rural and remote communities gain access to expertise that would otherwise be unavailable.
- **Cost efficiency**: AI reduces the burden on overstretched healthcare systems by automating preliminary assessments.
- **Scalable care**: One doctor can oversee hundreds of patients with AI handling routine monitoring and alerts.
- **Disaster response**: In emergencies, AI-powered mobile units can provide rapid triage and connect victims to remote specialists.

Challenges of AI in Global Telemedicine

- **Infrastructure**: Reliable internet, electricity, and digital literacy remain barriers in low-resource areas.
- **Regulation and licensing**: Telemedicine often crosses borders, raising legal and jurisdictional questions.
- **Equity in AI models**: Algorithms must be trained on diverse datasets to avoid bias that disadvantages underrepresented populations.
- **Trust**: Patients and providers need confidence that AI is reliable and secure.

Takeaway

AI-augmented telemedicine is one of the most promising tools for advancing global health equity. By automating triage, enhancing diagnostics, and enabling remote monitoring, AI helps deliver quality care to communities that need it most. While infrastructure and policy challenges remain, the trend is clear: the future of healthcare is not limited to hospitals in wealthy cities—it is digital, distributed, and global.

Building Trust Between Humans and AI Systems

AI in healthcare offers extraordinary potential—faster diagnoses, personalized treatment, and expanded global access. Yet, its success depends on one critical factor: **trust**. Patients must trust that AI is safe, fair, and private. Clinicians must trust that AI complements their expertise rather than undermines it. Without this trust, even the most advanced systems risk rejection. Building confidence between humans and AI is therefore as important as technological innovation itself.

Why Trust Matters

Healthcare is inherently personal. Patients share sensitive information, place their well-being in the hands of professionals, and expect accountability. Introducing AI adds new questions:

- Can I trust this system with my data?
- Is the AI making decisions fairly?
- Who is responsible if something goes wrong?

Trust is not automatic; it must be earned through transparency, reliability, and accountability.

Transparency and Explainability

One of the biggest challenges is the **black-box problem**—many AI systems produce results without showing how they reached them. In healthcare, this is unacceptable. Clinicians need to understand the reasoning behind AI recommendations before acting on them.

Solutions include:

- **Explainable AI (XAI)**: Models designed to show which features influenced their decision (e.g., highlighting suspicious areas on an X-ray).
- **Clear communication**: Providing patients with understandable explanations of how AI contributes to their care.
- **Auditability**: Keeping records of AI decision-making processes for review.

Reliability and Validation

Trust grows when AI consistently delivers accurate results across diverse settings. This requires:

- **Rigorous testing** before deployment, with large, diverse datasets.
- **Independent validation** by regulators and clinical institutions.
- **Continuous monitoring** after rollout, ensuring the system adapts to changing patient populations.

For example, if an AI model for cancer detection is validated across multiple hospitals worldwide, clinicians and patients alike will have greater confidence in its recommendations.

Human–AI Collaboration

AI should not be seen as replacing doctors but as **augmenting human expertise**. Trust improves when:

- Clinicians remain the ultimate decision-makers.
- AI is framed as a tool for support, not substitution.
- Patients are reassured that their care is guided by humans, with AI providing additional insight.

This "human-in-the-loop" model ensures accountability while maximizing the strengths of both AI and medical professionals.

Ethical and Regulatory Safeguards

Regulation also plays a role in building trust. Patients and providers need assurance that:

- Data privacy is protected under laws like HIPAA and GDPR.
- AI systems meet approved safety and fairness standards.
- Liability is clearly defined if errors occur.

Ethical frameworks must ensure that AI respects dignity, fairness, and human rights—values that technology alone cannot guarantee.

Takeaway

Building trust in AI healthcare is about more than accuracy—it requires transparency, reliability, fairness, and clear human oversight. When patients feel their data is safe and their care remains human-centered, and when clinicians feel AI enhances rather than threatens their expertise, adoption will grow. Trust is the foundation of the future of AI in medicine—and without it, innovation will remain unused potential.

Preparing Healthcare Professionals for the AI Era

The rise of AI in healthcare is not only a technological shift—it is a cultural and professional transformation. Doctors, nurses, researchers, and administrators will increasingly work alongside intelligent systems. To make the most of these tools, healthcare professionals must be prepared with new skills, new ways of thinking, and a willingness to adapt. Preparing the workforce is just as critical as building the technology itself.

Why Preparation Is Essential

AI adoption can succeed or fail depending on how clinicians engage with it. Without preparation:

- Doctors may distrust or ignore AI tools.
- Nurses and technicians may feel overwhelmed by new systems.
- Institutions may face wasted investments if tools are underused.

With preparation, however, AI becomes a **partner**—reducing workload, guiding better decisions, and expanding care.

New Skills for the AI Era

Healthcare professionals will not need to become programmers, but they will need **AI literacy**. This includes:

- **Understanding AI capabilities and limits**: Knowing what AI can and cannot do prevents both over-reliance and skepticism.
- **Interpreting AI outputs**: Clinicians must learn to critically evaluate AI recommendations in context.
- **Data awareness**: Professionals need to understand how data quality, diversity, and bias affect AI performance.
- **Digital communication**: As telemedicine and AI assistants expand, clinicians must develop new ways to engage with patients through digital platforms.

AI training should be integrated into medical and nursing education, ensuring the next generation is fluent in working with these tools.

Human–AI Collaboration in Practice

The most effective healthcare will come from **human–AI teams**. Professionals must learn when to rely on AI insights and when to override them with clinical judgment. For example:

- A radiologist may use AI to highlight suspicious areas in an MRI but still makes the final interpretation.
- A primary care doctor may use AI to predict diabetes risk but adjusts recommendations based on lifestyle discussions with the patient.

Training programs should emphasize this **collaborative mindset—** AI as an assistant, not a replacement.

Addressing Fears and Resistance

Some clinicians fear that AI will replace them or devalue their expertise. Preparing professionals for the AI era also means addressing these concerns:

- **Reassurance**: AI reduces administrative burdens and supports decision-making but cannot replace empathy, ethical judgment, or complex reasoning.
- **Involvement**: Clinicians should be part of AI system design, ensuring tools fit real-world workflows.
- **Continuous support**: Ongoing training and feedback ensure smooth adoption, rather than overwhelming staff with sudden change.

Institutional Responsibility

Hospitals and healthcare organizations must invest in:

- **Training programs** for current staff.
- **AI ethics education** to ensure responsible use.
- **Interdisciplinary teams** where clinicians, data scientists, and engineers collaborate.
- **Supportive policies** that encourage experimentation while safeguarding patient safety.

The burden of preparation should not fall on individuals alone—it is a shared responsibility across institutions and regulators.

Takeaway

Preparing healthcare professionals for the AI era means more than technical training. It requires cultivating trust, fostering collaboration, and empowering clinicians to use AI as a tool that enhances their expertise. With proper preparation, the future of healthcare will not be AI replacing humans but **humans and AI working together**, delivering safer, smarter, and more compassionate care.

Glossary

Adversarial Attack
A method of manipulating AI systems by subtly altering input data (like an image) so the algorithm misclassifies it, often without humans noticing.

Algorithm
A set of rules or instructions used by computers to process data and solve problems. In healthcare, algorithms can predict disease risk, interpret scans, or suggest treatments.

Artificial Intelligence (AI)
The simulation of human intelligence by machines, allowing them to perform tasks such as learning, reasoning, and problem-solving.

Augmented Reality (AR)
Technology that overlays digital information onto the real world, often used in medical training or surgery to enhance visualization.

Bias (AI Bias)
Systematic errors in AI models caused by unbalanced or incomplete training data, leading to unfair or inaccurate outcomes for certain groups.

Black-Box Model
An AI system that produces results without showing how it reached them, making its decision-making process difficult to interpret.

Clinical Decision Support (CDS)
AI tools that assist healthcare providers by analyzing patient data and offering evidence-based recommendations.

Clinical Trial
A research study conducted with human participants to test the safety and effectiveness of new drugs, treatments, or devices.

Computer Vision
An AI field that enables machines to "see" and interpret images, widely used in radiology and pathology.

Cybersecurity
The practice of protecting digital systems and data from unauthorized access, attacks, or theft.

Data Anonymization
The process of removing personal identifiers from datasets to protect patient privacy while allowing analysis.

Deep Learning
A type of machine learning using neural networks with many layers to analyze complex data such as medical images or speech.

Digital Twin
A virtual replica of a patient, organ, or system that can simulate medical conditions and predict outcomes.

Electronic Health Record (EHR)
A digital version of a patient's medical history, including diagnoses, treatments, lab results, and imaging.

Explainable AI (XAI)
AI designed to make its reasoning transparent, helping clinicians understand why specific predictions or recommendations were made.

Federated Learning
A privacy-preserving AI method where algorithms are trained across multiple institutions without transferring raw patient data.

General Data Protection Regulation (GDPR)
A European Union law that regulates the collection, storage, and use of personal data, including medical information.

Genomics
The study of an individual's complete set of DNA (genome), often used in personalized medicine.

Health Insurance Portability and Accountability Act (HIPAA)
A U.S. law that protects patient health information and governs how it can be shared and stored.

Machine Learning (ML)
A subset of AI where algorithms learn patterns from data without explicit programming, improving their performance over time.

Metaverse Medicine
The use of immersive virtual environments (VR/AR) for healthcare applications, including training, telemedicine, and patient education.

Molecular Simulation
AI-assisted modeling of how molecules (like drugs) interact with biological targets, accelerating drug discovery.

Natural Language Processing (NLP)
AI that enables computers to understand and analyze human language, used to interpret clinical notes and patient records.

Neural Network
A computational system inspired by the human brain, made up of layers of interconnected nodes that process data and detect patterns.

Predictive Analytics
The use of AI and statistical models to forecast future health outcomes, such as disease risk or treatment success.

Precision Medicine
A medical approach that tailors treatment to the individual based on genetics, lifestyle, and other personal factors.

Robotics in Healthcare
AI-driven machines used for surgery, rehabilitation, caregiving, and hospital logistics.

Telemedicine
The delivery of healthcare services remotely using telecommunications technology, often enhanced by AI.

Wearables
Devices like smartwatches or sensors that continuously collect health data such as heart rate, sleep, or glucose levels.

Thank You

Thank you for taking the time to read this book. My goal in writing *AI in Healthcare* was to make a complex, rapidly evolving topic clear, practical, and accessible for everyone—whether you are a healthcare professional, a student, or simply curious about the future of medicine.

If this book has helped you better understand the opportunities and challenges of AI in healthcare, then it has served its purpose.

Books like this reach more readers when people like you share your feedback. If you found value in these pages, I would be deeply grateful if you could take a moment to leave an honest review on **Amazon**. Reviews not only help others decide if the book is right for them, but they also support the continued creation of straightforward, easy-to-read guides like this one.

Your thoughts matter—and your voice helps this knowledge reach the people who need it most.

With gratitude,
Eric LeBouthillier

www.ingramcontent.com/pod-product-compliance
Lightning Source LLC
Chambersburg PA
CBHW071714210326
41597CB00017B/2484